Talking About Death Won't Kill You

The Essential Guide To End-Of-Life Conversations

Dr. Kathy Kortes-Miller

16
EasyRead Large

RHYW

Copyright Page from the Original Book

Published by ECW Press
665 Gerrard Street East
Toronto, Ontario, Canada M4M 1Y2
416-694-3348 / info@ecwpress.com

Editor for the press: Susan Renouf
Cover design: David A. Gee
Author photo: Jessica L. Wyatt Photography

Library and Archives Canada Cataloguing in Publication

Kortes-Miller, Kathy, author
Talking about death won't kill you : the essential guide to end-of-life conversations / Dr. Kathy Kortes-Miller.

Includes bibliographical references and index.
Issued in print and electronic formats.
ISBN 978-1-77041-406-8 (softcover).
ALSO ISSUED AS: 978-1-77305-177-2 (PDF), 978-1-77305-176-5 (ePUB)

1. Death—Psychological aspects.
I. Title. II. Title: Talking about death will not kill you.

BF789.D4K67 2018 155.9'37
C2017-906595-5 C2017-906596-3

Printing: MARQUIS 5 4 3 2 1
PRINTED AND BOUND IN CANADA

The publication of *Talking About Death Won't Kill You* has been generously supported by the Government of Canada through the Canada Book Fund. *Ce livre est financé en partie par le gouvernement du Canada.* We also acknowledge the contribution of the Government of Ontario through the Ontario Book Publishing Tax Credit and the Ontario Media Development Corporation.

Ontario
Ontario Media Development Corporation

Canada

TABLE OF CONTENTS

For Derrick, who showed us how to live, laugh and love well And Shirley, who will always love him

INTRODUCTION

Why Dying Matters to Me

"There may be no single thing that can teach us more about life than death."
—Arianna Huffington

I remember clearly the very first day of my second shot at a Ph.D. program. I sat in a circle with my fellow new students. It felt a bit like kindergarten, but it was exciting nonetheless. There we were, all of us eager to divulge our plans for research and how we hoped to make a difference in the world. One by one, we shared our ideas and passions and talked about what we wanted to study and why. Our peers responded enthusiastically, nodding their heads, asking questions and making suggestions for further reading, other scholars and researchers to explore. It felt like a supportive, collaborative space.

When it was my turn, I leaned forward into this great group of people and said, "I want to study death education."

There was silence in the room. Crickets.

Finally, after what felt like an uncomfortably long pause, one of the professors—a seemingly kind and gentle soul—spoke up. "Ahhh," he said. "Deaf education. So, you want to work with the hearing-impaired?"

"Uh, no, not really," I replied, trying to push down a sense of dread and panic. "I'm thinking death ... with a 'th.'"

Silence.

"As in dying, dead, death," I stammered.

More crickets.

That's when it occurred to me that maybe we're all a bit hard of hearing when it comes to talking about the end of life.

This reception to my research idea was a bit disheartening. Here I was, proposing to focus exhaustively for the next five or more years on a subject that no one wanted to talk about. I might have considered finding a new topic, giving up on death. But I knew I couldn't. That's because I'd already had the experience of being shut down when I'd tried to talk about dying. And I was determined not to let it happen again.

The previous year, precisely 12 days before I was to start that same Ph.D. program, I was diagnosed with cancer. I was 37, a mother of two active children, a wife and an educator, and I had a malignant tumour, 10 centimetres long, in my colon. Instead of beginning my studies, I spent a year in treatment, putting on hold not only the Ph.D. but most aspects of my life as I recovered from my surgery and learned how to navigate what they call "the new normal."

After I was diagnosed, I was referred to a very well-respected surgeon, considered one of the best in her field in Canada. We met on the day I was supposed to begin my first Ph.D. course. I wanted to tell this surgeon that I was scared. I wanted to tell her I was afraid of dying and leaving my children without their mother. I wanted to tell her what I really should have been doing that day instead and how heartbroken—and, frankly, pissed off—I was to be in her office rather than at school!

But I didn't get the chance to say any of those things. "If you're going to get cancer, this is the kind to get," the surgeon told me matter-of-factly. I was a bit confused: I had just told her that my aunt had died of the same disease when she was only a few years older than I. Still, I managed to get up the guts to say, "I'm really scared I'm going to die, and there are some things I want you to know."

She shut me down. "Don't talk like that," she said. "You are not going to die."

And, you know, she was right. Thank God, she was right. I haven't died yet! I owe that surgeon a debt of gratitude for her role in saving my life. Still, though, I wished then, as I wished throughout my treatment, and as I wish now, that someone—one of the multitude of health-care providers I encountered throughout my time as a cancer patient—would have talked with me about the "death elephant" in the room. I could have died. My aunt did. Many others have. I'd supported some of them. I needed someone to hear me out, to let me take ownership of my living until I died.

That's what I want for all of us: to feel like we have a sense of control, to feel heard and to feel safe to talk about dying and death in the midst of our life and living. I want us to have a better death education.

Your Death Education

Take a moment to think about your own death education: How have you learned and how do you continue to learn about dying and death? What was your first lesson? Who was your teacher? What was your take-home message? And how does the sum total of your death education thus far serve you today in how you think and talk about dying and death?

If you're shrugging your shoulders and shaking your head in puzzlement (My "death education"? Who has a death education?) at my questions, you're not alone. Most of us spend more time choosing a new car than we do thinking about the end of life. The vast majority of us have very little in the way of formal (not to mention informal) training or education about what it means to die. I teach an undergraduate course to future health-care providers—called Introduction to Palliative Care—about how to support people who are dying. Most of the 18- and 19-year-olds who take my course have never experienced the death of someone close to them and have thought very little, if at all, about what death means to them. This isn't unusual: the average health-care professional receives only a few hours of death education over the course of his or her schooling, if they are lucky. If our front-line medical workers, the very people who will most often confront death and dying, have so little in the way of death education, how can they properly and compassionately and productively care for people who are dying? And how can the rest of us, without any formal training, hope to do the same? Let alone think about what we might want for ourselves.

No wonder we struggle with understanding death. Somehow, we've forgotten that we must face the end of our own lives and those of our loved ones. Let's face it: all of us will be intimate with death at least once. Yet we live in a death-denying and death-defying society. We try to pretend death doesn't exist. If someone we love dies, we are granted (or we grant ourselves) only a brief period to grieve, to mourn, and then the expectations of life kick us right back into overdrive. We are expected to get on with things, get over the person we lost—in no small part to make things easier for those around us. I returned to working with people who were dying three days after my aunt, with whom I was very close, died.

This approach does not serve us well. It creates a vicious cycle: we neglect our death education (it's easy to do when no one ever brings up the topic or offers us a course), so we lack the emotional and practical skills when it comes to facing death. Because we tend to fear what we don't know, we become increasingly scared of talking openly about the end of life. Complicating this is the fact that most of us already fear the process of dying: we're scared about pain, loss of control, losing people we love, being ripped from our own lives, uncertainty. That fear can lead to anger as we pretend that dying and death aren't integral parts of life and living. We feel isolated as we grapple alone, trying to make sense of our emotions around death. Many of us feel ashamed: of our fears, of our lack of knowledge—even of our desire to learn more about the end of life. All these negative emotions can lead to denial; we'd rather not experience them, so we work even harder to avoid learning about death. And then, when we're faced with death—with the cancer diagnosis or the progressive disease or the car accident or the eventual decline of old age—we are too overcome with grief, disbelief and denial to think about and plan for it coherently.

We need to break this cycle.

When we do break it, we become open to learning and talking about dying and death as a part of life. In so doing, we can change the conversation from something negative to one of understanding, compassion and acceptance. Our newly developed and healthy respect for dying and death will strengthen us on both personal and societal levels. We will be able to take better care of our dying and approach our own deaths with less fear and more comfort. When we demystify death and encourage critical thinking, research and debate about it, we will better learn how to support one another in this unavoidable part of life. And we need to begin this work before we, or our loved ones, get sick and before we become overcome by grief, fear and denial. We have to start today to develop our knowledge and understanding and to shift our thinking.

We can do this. We've already done it, ironically, with the beginning of life: birth. In only a couple of generations, we have greatly transformed childbirth from a highly medicalized, mysterious, doctor-centric and sometimes shameful or embarrassing process into one that puts mothers, babies and parents at the centre. We have hundreds of books and countless websites and forums devoted to pregnancy and birth. We talk about it constantly and, more often than not, women have at least some say in how, when and where they will give birth and who will help them do so. New mothers report feeling empowered because they had the opportunity to make plans, learn about the birthing process and share stories with other women. I'm not arguing here that we have perfected childbirth in the Western world, but it is normal (and advantageous) to talk openly and often about how we would like our babies to be born.

Now we need to do the same with dying. In the same way that we increasingly understand birth as a social and natural—rather than a medical—process, we need to understand death as a human experience, as social as birth and as worthy of our attention, education and conversation. We need the same kind of research into the benefits of comprehensive death education. We do know that when people feel empowered to talk about their dying, and feel supported and cared for at the end of their lives, they report having less fear, less pain and less anxiety. Those close to the dying person—and each death has a direct impact on at least five people—report that the dying process is meaningful and provides an opportunity to discuss unfinished business, hopes and dreams, and to say good-bye. When we believe that how we die matters, we are more likely to make plans, have important conversations and ultimately die with less regret. We will still grieve our losses, but we will also find solace in knowing that our loved ones died with a sense of control and that they were well cared for. It is the same for our own deaths; we will have a sense of closure and control, and we will hopefully have made peace with the paths our lives have taken.

As Dame Cicely Saunders, the founder of the modern Hospice Palliative movement, said, "How people die remains in the memory of those who live on." The way we care for people at the end of life reflects our values and compassion as a society.

Changing our approach to death requires a shift not only in our own attitudes but also in our medical establishment. Death is inevitable; it is rarely a medical "failure." But our medical system is trained to "fix" things. That's great when what ails you is fixable, but not everything is. As palliative care physician and author Dr. Ira Byock writes, "Our health-care system is well-honed to fight disease, but poorly designed to meet the basic needs of seriously ill and dying patients and their families. We can do both. We must." We need to find space in our medical and health-care systems to allow natural death. We cannot continue to abandon people when medicine can't cure them, to tell them "there's nothing more we can do."

Because we can do lots to prepare for dying. And it starts with talking about it. It extends to creating communities that step up in a compassionate way when we need them. I think we're ready: the Canadian Hospice Palliative Care Association reported in 2014 that nearly three-quarters of Canadians are beginning to think about the end of life.

Perhaps I am selfish, but now, when as I teach, I imagine the students in my courses as one day being charged with caring for me at the end of my life. I try to instill in them a desire to connect with people, separate from their diseases or conditions. I challenge them to recognize that learning with their heart is a part of their education that needs to be nurtured and developed every bit as much as their clinical skills and theoretical knowledge. I encourage them to think about how they will want to be cared for when they are dying. Ratner and Song (2002) speak to an overarching goal for comprehensive death education that resonates with me: "As educators, we claim to prepare our students for life. We need to prepare them for death as well."

I know that talking about death isn't easy: it is sad and scary, and—for many—it's a taboo topic. I've had to do it as a healthcare provider, fumbling through conversations as I learned on the job. More recently, I have had to do it as a patient, a friend, a wife, a daughter and a mother. But for me, it is essential. We need to bring death out into the open, witness it, talk about it, learn about it and recognize that dying matters because it is an inevitable part of our lives. And in so doing, we can be more prepared, make better decisions about the kind of care we want and ultimately improve the dying experience for ourselves and those we love. I now know that when I am dying, I want to be cared for by people who do not avoid the elephant in the room—the reality of death. I need those closest to me to believe that dying matters.

So, I bet today isn't a good day for you to die. Hopefully tomorrow won't be, either. But maybe today is a good day for you to start talking about death. Let's take death out of the closet and give ourselves—and those we love—a gift and make space in our living for our dying. Canadians are going to be talking about dying and death a lot over the next few years as baby boomers age, and as we figure out how to move forward in light of the Supreme Court of Canada's decisions regarding medically hastened death, which I explore in detail in Chapter 9.

We owe it to our families, friends and communities to show them that dying matters.

We owe it to one of the first patients I ever cared for, who told me in no uncertain terms that she was too young to die, but everyone treated her like she was too old to live. She was 94.

We owe it to the children we confuse when we use euphemisms to talk about dying and death ("Grandma's gone"; "We put the dog to sleep"), instead of clear, honest language to explain this important life event.

We owe it to the groups of tweens/teens who sit in the dark in movie theatres and sob when their beloved characters, like Augustus in *The Fault in Our Stars,* die. We cannot let movies and books do all the teaching about death for us. We need to talk to our children about dying in the light of day.

We owe it to the vast majority of Canadians (anywhere from 70 to 84 percent) who, according to the Canadian Hospice Palliative Care Association, do not have access to palliative and end-of-life care services, and to even more Canadians who have no access to grief and bereavement services. We need to make death education and these services more accessible to all.

We owe it to the First Nations, who are working hard to figure out how to provide palliative and end-of-life care for elders in their own communities, in ways that honour their traditions.

We owe it to those who phone the call-in radio shows on euthanasia and assisted death and tell us that we treat animals better than humans because at least we euthanize our pets when they are old, sick and in pain.

We owe it to our health-care providers, who are just beginning to figure out that allowing natural death is not a failure, and who are learning how to integrate, when it's appropriate, hospice palliative care.

We owe it to the baby boomers, who are going to let us know exactly what they expect from us at the end of their lives.

And we owe it to my friend Derrick. Exactly one year ago, two weeks before he turned 50, Derrick was diagnosed with acute myeloid leukemia, an aggressive form of cancer in the blood. He has spent the past 12 months fighting his cancer—rounds of chemotherapy and radiation that left him nauseated, weak and hairless; a stem cell transplant that isolated him from his friends and home; and experimental treatments that offered a shred of hope. I remember the day he learned that that last hope for a cure failed: his cancer was back. Derrick is dying. He may have only weeks left to live.

When I walked into his hospital room, Derrick looked beaten and exhausted. He reminded me of a fighter who realized he has lost his battle. We hugged. We cried. And he said to me, "I need to talk to you about dying."

Derrick didn't talk much about dying while he was fighting for his life. In some ways, he couldn't: just getting through his treatment took all his strength and energy. Today, though, he had questions about what the rest of his life might look like. He wanted us to know what is important to him now: time with his family and friends. He was scared and worried about how his death will affect those he loves. What will his wife do? They had always assumed she would die first. What kind of plans does he need to make? Derrick was tired of being in the hospital; he wanted to be at home. Would this be possible? He was worried about how his dying would affect my young son, who calls Derrick his best friend. This is only the first of many hard and important conversations we will have.

I wish with all my heart that this wasn't happening to my friend. But I'm so very grateful that I am equipped to talk about dying with him. How Derrick dies matters. It matters because his death will affect his family, friends and community. It matters because he is my close friend and I love him dearly. Although I would much rather be helping him plan his next holiday or home renovation project, I'm honoured that he trusts me enough to talk about his death with me.

I know I need to be a sounding board for his questions and a safe place for his fears and strong emotions. I am indebted to all those individuals who have taught me the importance of these conversations: medical professionals and spiritual leaders, and—most importantly—individuals facing death themselves.

And this is what I want this book to offer readers: a chance to reflect, to learn how to support, to be present and to engage in meaningful conversations so that when the time comes, we will all be prepared to show our loved one that dying matters.

How to Use This Book

Before we delve further into our conversations about how and why dying and death are an important part of life, I'd like to clarify what this book is and what it is not.

It is my profound hope that it will galvanize you, the reader, to recognize that dying and death are an integral part of life and living, and that by learning about it and talking about it, you and those you love will ultimately live fuller lives. I want this book to be a catalyst for change in the conversations you have with those most important to you and with your health-care providers. I appreciate that these conversations are not easy, but I know that they are worth the effort.

This book is not prescriptive. It is not a to-do list that must be completed before you die. I'm not here to tell you what to do or what decisions you need to make. Rather, I am here to support you in a process that will empower you to begin to figure out some of these things for yourself. The questions posed in this book are designed to do just that. The stories shared are not to demonstrate any right or wrong way. They are here to act as a stimulus for further discussion and reflection. Each and every one of us will face the end of our own and our loved ones' lives uniquely, as we discover what works for us and those we care about.

It is my dearest hope that this book will change the way you think about dying and death, and may help you to make the dying process more meaningful and gentler for yourself or for someone you love.

CHAPTER ONE

Why Dying Matters

"Learn as if you were going to live forever. Live as if you were going to die tomorrow."
—Author unknown

"I cannot pretend I am without fear. But my predominant feeling is one of gratitude."
—Oliver Sacks, a British neurologist, on his own experience with dying

Cutting to the Chase

I am going to die. You are going to die. Everyone is going to die. To paraphrase the inimitable John Cleese, "Life is a terminal illness that is sexually transmitted." We are born to die. But somewhere along the way, we manage to forget that *death is a part of life.* From the moment of our birth, our cells are already dying. We are always experiencing cellular death; we are always dying. It is time to acknowledge that talking and thinking about death will not kill us; we need to stop denying its existence.

This book is designed to get you talking about that elephant in the room: dying and death. Most of us dread these conversations and run from them. For many of us, talking about dying and death is taboo and much too difficult. I invite you to use this book to begin to think and reflect on dying and death, and in so doing, find it less overwhelming or unnerving. It is my hope that you will reflect on your own living, and how you want the end of your life to look. And that by doing this, you can open conversation with your loved ones about what they want for their end of life. If you are a medical professional, thinking about what you want for yourself will help you talk with the people you provide care for.

Engaging in this kind of reflection and thinking will allow you to embrace life more fully, and with less fear and trepidation. Who doesn't want that?

Death Denial and Death Ignorance

How did dying and death become something we all know will happen to each and every one of us, but that we try to avoid discussing? If death is part of the total human experience, how is it that we spend so much time and energy thinking about anything else? Many have said that we live in a death-denying and death-defying society.

But to saying this may be an oversimplification. Death does intrude—often rudely—on our lives and thoughts. It cannot be denied. It is the ultimate form of human vulnerability, regardless of who we are, what we know, whom we know or what we own. It will happen to us all; it is intrinsic to the human condition and connected with how we live. To better understand why we think about dying and death the way we do today, we must understand the role it has played in Western history.

How We Used to Die

The experience of death varies from culture to culture and from era to era. Until the mid-twentieth century, death was considered to be a natural and inevitable part of the lives of North Americans and Europeans. Infectious diseases such as smallpox, tuberculosis and influenza were constant concerns. Accidents were common and wars were pretty much endemic. Life expectancy was significantly lower than it is today. Dying and death were familiar because they were visible. Women and babies died regularly in childbirth. Children sometimes went without names for up to a year until it was determined that they had a good chance of survival. A tough existence, great risk of infection, lower standards of living, poor sanitation, lack of medicines—these factors all contributed to a lower life expectancy. Dying typically involved signs and symptoms that people recognized, such as diarrhea, vomiting, headache, muscle pain or laboured breathing. People were exposed to enough dying and death that they recognized when people were seriously ill. They were well-acquainted with death because it was a frequent occurrence in their lives.

Because death was a routine part of life and hospitalization was less common, the dying were primarily cared for by their families and communities. That care was largely supportive—there was usually little they could do medically—to ensure that loved ones were made as comfortable as possible. Families and communities provided care, including a place to rest, shelter from the elements, cold compresses and nurturing food (if the individual who was ill could eat or drink). Spiritual intercession such as prayer, song and support from religious representatives played a major role.

People usually died in their homes. Friends and family prepared the body for burial, and it was laid out in the best room of the house so that people could pay their respects. Friends and loved ones kept a vigil, drinking tea (or more) and eating sandwiches, chatting, weeping and laughing. Children learned early that this was what death looked like, and that it was normal, if puzzling.

With advancements in our understanding of disease and sanitation, life expectancy in North America and some parts of Europe began to increase in the early 1900s. These changes were primarily because of the improvements in the standard of living initiated by the public-health movement. Over time, the movement reduced the incidence and severity of many illnesses, infections and other common health ailments. A more modern approach to health care focused on sanitation and decreasing the transmission of infectious diseases.

Treatment and public education supplied by doctors and nurses also improved maternal and child health. There was a shift from acute death-causing diseases to more chronic conditions, such as arthritis, heart disease and diabetes, that affected the quality of one's life.

Hospitals also became more common, often run by charitable institutions. They were large, crowded and unpleasant places filled with people who had a variety of different and potentially contagious ailments. This resulted in the hospitals themselves sometimes being life-threatening. It was in these hospitals, however, that nurses and doctors learned skills and developed knowledge about disease, surgery and infection control as they worked to ward off illness and death. People began to live longer.

With this increase in life expectancy and the shift from acute illness to more chronic conditions, the focus of health-care systems also changed—from disease management to prolonging life. Our health-care system made some spectacular advances, such as developing surgical procedures to repair and replace essential organs and functions and inventing artificial support systems such as feeding tubes and ventilators to prolong life. With all these advances in sanitation and disease control, people began to live well significantly longer. They not only lived longer; they expected to live longer. There was a paradigm shift from dying being an anticipated, familiar part of living to it becoming remote and expected only in old age.

How We Die Today

Over the past 150 years, how we view death has been informed and influenced by these advances in science and medicine. Science has found cures for many previously untreatable diseases and ailments while modern medicine has managed to successfully limit the effects of many previously fatal diseases. Families no longer feel compelled to have large numbers of children because they are concerned that many of them will not live past childhood.

Many of the illnesses that were once consistently terminal no longer result in immediate death following a diagnosis. More often than not, the individual is on a trajectory that may include both improvements and declines in health. Current health-care treatment includes interventions that aim to prolong and maintain life. Often a person can survive a life-threatening illness for up to 15 years, or even more. In the past, that same illness would have caused a quick death. In most places in North America, a death is considered premature if it occurs in an individual before age 75. In 2012, in Canada, the average age at death was 81 years of age.

Sometimes death is instant, from a massive injury or stroke, for example, but more often the dying process will take days or weeks as the person's condition deteriorates. Regardless of the type of death, we expect that while we may need or want to pitch in when a loved one is dying at home, our heath-care system will provide treatment as his or her death becomes imminent.

Because most deaths now occur in old age and generally as a result of a chronic health condition, such as heart disease or cancer, we are also older than previous generations when we have our first personal experience of death. In Introduction to Palliative Care, my entry-level course about caring for people who are dying, it is becoming more common for my 19- and 20-year-old students never to have experienced the death of someone close to them.

The advances in health care over the past century are exciting and life-extending, but they have left us with some challenges we now need to face. Medicine presents us with more choices and decisions than ever before about how and when we will die. We are often required to make these life-and-death decisions rapidly, and they often involve concepts and language that are entirely unfamiliar. As well, because of these advances many people who might have at one time died in the familiar surroundings of their home with their loved ones beside them are now institutionalized and cared for by paid professionals who do not know them the way their family and friends might. This has allowed the rest of us to distance ourselves from the later stages of life. Some families report feeling compelled to leave the care of their dying loved one solely to the professionals, who are seen as knowing more about what should be done.

The ability of medicine and modern technology to prolong life has sometimes caused the process of dying to be perceived as more terrifying than death itself. In our attempts to defy death and prolong life, we will try anything. Some people find themselves or their loved ones hooked up to life-support machines that are capable of keeping them alive physically but in a state that is sorely lacking in quality or meaning. Sometimes people will agree to treatments or surgeries that are more painful and debilitating than the disease itself. Our newfound capabilities have raised numerous issues about autonomy and who has the right to choose how and when we die. Who has the right to decide when someone may discontinue life support? Refuse treatment? Allow for a natural death? Often, we find ourselves in unfamiliar territory, overwhelmed with grief and unequipped to make the required decisions when our loved ones are at this critical juncture. Or we are as overwhelmed as our families by decisions about how we wish to be treated in our last days if it is our own death we face. It is imperative that we reverse this trend. We need to talk with one another about what matters to us, what we dream of and hope for, so that when the time comes, we will know how to make the decisions that are right for us, and so that we know the wishes of our loved ones.

Social and Cultural Responses to Dying and Death

Yes, we have made incredible medical advances, but we must remember that dying and death are not always, or only, medical events. Perhaps more important, death is also a *social* process. It is vital to recognize the roles social networks, communities and cultures have played in our understanding of dying. In his book *How We Die,* Dr. Sherwin Nuland states that "death belongs to the dying and to those who love them." It would be wonderful if this were true. And although many people and organizations advocate for this, we are not there yet. The current national sociocultural climate demonstrates that the majority of Canadians wish to improve the care of the dying, or to have more options for end-of-life care. Three-quarters (74 percent) of Canadians report having thought about how they would like to be cared for at the end of their lives. Most Canadians, when asked, report that they would like to die at home, yet 70 percent of deaths occur in hospitals (CHPCA, 2014).

Dr. Ira Byock, an author and physician specializing in palliative care, has observed that we can learn a lot about a society by seeking to understand how it deals with death and how it cares for those who are nearing the end of their lives. In our new, technologically advanced world we have developed a view of death as a failure. We make statements like "The patient failed treatment." We have isolated the event to the point where it is rarely seen in our communities. Elderly family members often spend their last days in nursing homes, hospitals or extended-care facilities. As a result, most family members are not active, physical or hands-on care-providers in their loved ones' dying process, and they are no longer learning about dying and death through the provision of care in the home. The philosopher Philippe Ariès, a pioneer in the study of attitudes toward childhood and death, calls this "Invisible Death." Ariès recognized that in the 21st century, we spend our energy isolating ourselves from death, keeping it separate from our everyday selves. We make it invisible so that it does not interfere with our living.

Today, most people die in sterile hospital rooms with strict visiting hours, cared for by professionals. They find themselves in a strange and isolating environment, attached to tubes, wires and/or machines. They are frequently told to fight for their lives. Sometimes they will not even be told that they are dying for fear this will take away their hope and desire to fight. This attitude does not allow people the opportunity to prepare for their death, to resolve any "unfinished" business, such as saying good-bye and I love you. They miss out on the opportunity to maintain some autonomy, control and a sense of peace in their dying. They and their families miss out on the opportunity to participate in rituals associated with dying and death that might bring them comfort.

Social Rituals Honouring Death

Societies have always used rituals that teach people how to act after another has died. These rituals have taught us what to wear, what to say, what to do with the body, and how to care for those who are grieving. There is archeological evidence of death rituals that date back to the Neanderthals, more than 150,000 years ago. Archeologists have found decorated shells, tools, animal antlers and other objects next to corpses, indicating that there was some sort of ritual performed after the death. And throughout history, post-death rituals have been used to protect the living or to ensure that the spirit of the individual who died transitions safely to wherever it may be going. Our rituals may change with time and culture, but the sentiment remains. We wish to respect the dead and comfort the living.

In smaller communities where I've worked, the townspeople use simple rituals to show that they care for the people who have experienced the death of a loved one. After a death, families would talk about expecting the "casserole brigade" and the need to make sure there was space in the freezer for all the incoming food that would mean they didn't have to think about shopping and cooking in the middle of their grieving. Nurturing others with food is one way that a community can demonstrate that they care.

I remember when my Greek grandfather died and my French grandmother, his much younger wife, was told in no uncertain terms that she needed to wear black for the 40 days that she would be mourning. I had never seen my grandmother wear black before, and she did not agree to this Greek tradition easily. But eventually she gave in begrudgingly. On the 40th day after his death, my Greek family threw a big party with tons of food, and many from the extended Greek community came to celebrate my grandfather's life. My grandmother, who had fought wearing black for a good part of the ritual period, told me she had decided to continue wearing black longer, as she had realized that it helped people understand that she was still grieving the death of her husband. She also said that participating in the ritual had made her feel connected to him.

Until quite recently in the 21st century, rituals such as the ones my Greek family practised were well-accepted. People followed them because they provided guidance on what to do after someone died, and communities were more homogeneous, united by heritage and religion. Now, however, these rituals and traditions that guided our actions and feelings around dying and death are changing. We are more diverse and some of us are less overtly religious. Our families often live at great distances. These factors may require new ways of honouring a death and celebrating a life. Some are even moving away from an immediate traditional funeral ritual or ceremony because many people find the expense too great, or the logistics of gathering together people who live in far-flung places too difficult. A celebration of life might happen long after the body has been buried or cremated and it adds to our distancing from death itself.

Getting Comfortable with Death

Even though we will all become familiar with at least one death in our lives, society does not recognize it as a normal part of our lives. On one hand, we try to avoid it at all costs, and on the other, it's in our face every time we turn on the TV. It's on the news and in our books, movies and music. We work to convince ourselves that it happens to other people—not us and those we love. This hiding of dying and death is ironic for those of us who have turned on the television lately. The dying and death we will be reflecting on in this book is not the kind you see on TV: there are no vampires or zombies; it does not happen halfway around the world. The kind of dying and death that our news and media show is not the kind of dying that the majority of North Americans will experience. The dying that we need to be discussing is the kind that happens to those we love and that will one day happen to us, too. We need to determine what dying and death mean to us, in our lives.

Dr. Richard Kalish, author of "The Social Context of Death and Dying," identifies three different meanings of death in our society:

- Death is an organizer of time. Time takes on a greater significance as our death grows closer, and as people begin to recognize that certain things may be happening for the very last time—for example, the last visit home, the last meal, the final time getting out of bed. How people measure time may also change when a person is dying. Sometimes it is measured by changes in the person's condition that may signal death is close. In other instances, time may be measured by the important life events that they are still hopeful to see and participate in, for example, the birth of a long-awaited grandchild or one last Christmas celebration.
- Death is a transition or passage for those who believe in an afterlife or transformation. Many people, including First Nations groups, choose not to speak of dying and death. When an individual is dying, they refer to him or her as "transitioning" or going to the "next place." Again, our use of language demonstrates our values and beliefs around the process of dying and death.
- Death is a significant loss experience. It is pervasive, causing loss of body, mind, personhood, memories, hopes and dreams. Losses experienced when an individual is dying are not only their

personal losses, such as loss of independence, loss of health status or loss of control, but also the loss of their relationships to others. Often people talk about how hard and challenging it is to say good-bye to someone who is dying. Yet the person dying must say good-bye to each and every important relationship they have. Those losses are numerous and often very painful.

There is a lot we can do to prepare for death. And it starts with talking about our own dying and the dying of others. It extends to creating communities that care for one another and step up in a compassionate way when we need them. It only makes sense that we make space to talk about dying and death and support individuals who are dying. Elisabeth Kübler-Ross, in her seminal book *On Death and Dying,* which was instrumental in encouraging people to pay attention to individuals who are dying, offers three reasons we need to do this:

- People who are dying are still alive and often have unfinished business they want and need to address.
- We need to listen actively to people who are dying so that we can provide the kind of care they want and need.
- People who are dying, with all their fear, concerns, hopes and dreams, have lots to teach us about our shared humanity and the final stages of life.

The attitudes we hold about dying and death, and the knowledge we possess about these life events, are reflected in the language we use, the mass media to which we are exposed, and the music, literature and visual arts surrounding us. Many of us will find ourselves unprepared to cope with death's intrusion on our lives, as all too often we choose to ignore death until our "number is up," or someone near to us dies. But if we spend some time and energy thinking about dying and death when we are hale and competent, if we talk about it with those we love, we may find that through our examination of death we develop a greater understanding of and reverence for life.

An "Appropriate" Death

Over time, the idea of a "good" death has changed. In earlier times, it often meant that you got to die in bed at the end of your natural life, not cut short by war, famine or disease. But our lives are immeasurably different now, safe and largely prosperous as we are in the West. And the idea of a "good" death is difficult for many—we would argue that there is nothing "good" about death. Some people working in palliative care, therefore, have begun to reframe the concept of a "good" death to one that focuses on an "appropriate" death.

An "appropriate" death is one that aligns with how a person has lived. The dying process is consistent with one's life experiences, social interactions and coping style. For example, a person who valued a life of independence, relative seclusion and autonomy might well seek these conditions at the end of life as well. He or she would receive support and care that respected these choices as much as possible.

Joe, a man I had the privilege of meeting while I worked on the hospice unit, was an example of someone determined to die the way he lived. Joe had been financially challenged all his life and claimed that money just got in the way of his living. He found the hospice unit uncomfortable; it was too "fancy" for him. It was important to Joe that he go home to die. Joe's home was not a place I would have wanted to live in, but it was his and he had his community there to support him. Joe wanted to die as he had he lived.

Some factors to consider in an appropriate death include

- Maintaining a sense of identity and making decisions that are true to that identity
- Reducing fears and internal conflicts
- Reflecting on the life lived
- Support for important relationships
- Continuing to recognize the need for hope and plans

Once we have answered some of these questions for ourselves, we can use them as the underpinnings for an advance care plan we build for ourselves. And we can use them to help us have these difficult conversations with others so that they can make their end-of-life wishes known to us.

Change Is in the Air

Dr. Peter Saul suggests we need a movement called "Occupy Death" to break the taboo we have created around dying and death. We need to reclaim our dying. Unfortunately, we have a long way to go. Health-care providers and scientists are trained to think that it is their job to overcome death, and they do everything in their power to make it so. But no one can stave off death forever, and through this well-meant medicalization of the end of life, we have given up our autonomy to die where, how and with whom we would like. Instead, we allow our health-care providers, institutions, drug companies, policy-makers and insurance companies to take over. Our fear and societal avoidance of dying as an integral part of life have caused us to relinquish the control and ownership of our dying. We have forgotten how to make dying the logical extension of our living. We have blocked family members and loved ones from taking on challenging and decisive roles in our dying because we won't talk about it. We lack the courage and language to have these important conversations with those we love. The reality and impact of scientific advancements have created the opportunity for us to live longer and healthier than ever before, but we cannot remove death from the human experience.

Let's make space in our living for our dying right now. In the chapters ahead, you will develop the tools and language to speak up and out about death. I want to invite you now to begin to take ownership of where you currently are in your relationship with death. The questions that follow will assist you in beginning this process. Take a moment and ask yourself:

- How did you first learn about dying and death?
- Where were you?
- Who was with you?
- How old were you when you first began to develop an understanding of death?
- Who was your teacher?
- What was your take-home message from that experience?
- What did death mean to you then?
- What does death mean to you now?

Reflect on these questions; discuss them and share the stories they evoke with those closest to you. In so doing, you will begin to take ownership of living until you die. You will also encourage your family and those close to you to be more open about their own thoughts and wishes for their dying.

The Canadian rock group Trooper reminds us, "We're here for a good time, not a long time." Talking about death does not have to be awkward or uncomfortable, because these are anxieties, fears and doubts that all of us have in common. Let us set the bar high and acknowledge that our lives will improve when we talk about the tough stuff, when we talk about dying and death. Let us learn to live a life that demonstrates dying matters.

CHAPTER TWO

Improving Our Death Literacy and Informed Decisions

"What is a fear of living? It's being preeminently afraid of dying. It is not doing what you came here to do, out of timidity and spinelessness. The antidote is to take full responsibility for yourself—for the time you take up and the space you occupy. If you don't know what you're here to do, then just do some good."
—Maya Angelou

"No one has ever escaped it, and that is how it should be, because death is very likely the single best invention of life. It's life's change agent. It clears out the old to make space for the new."
—Steve Jobs

One of the first people I ever had the privilege of supporting in my hospice work was a spirited woman named Liz. On our first meeting, she informed me in no uncertain terms that she was too young to die. She was 94. Liz had had a long and full life of adventure and learning. But like most of us, she hadn't devoted time or thought to what she wanted for the end of her life. Of course, she had encountered dying and death in her 94 years, but only from afar. She told me, "I know lots about living well but nothing about how to die." Liz also told me that she felt like she was going on a big trip without a map and did not know what to expect. She had fears about the dying process but did not want to admit them to her children because she did not want to burden them. Liz was scared that she was unprepared to die and did not feel like she had any control over what was going to happen next.

And then there was Ellen, who was dying of cancer. When she was admitted to our hospice unit, she unceremoniously handed me a binder. "It's all here," Ellen said. "Let me know if you have questions, but please let me get on with my living. I probably don't have much time left." The binder had information on her disease, the kind of care she wanted, her thoughts about and direction for resuscitation, a list of whom to contact before she died, the location of her important documents, directions for funeral arrangements and even some suggestions for her obituary. This binder represented Ellen's efforts to get her affairs in order before she died. She had been a planner all her life, and was determined that her plans and her binder would guide her dying. Her health-care team had a few questions to ensure we were all on the same page, but for the most part we focused on making sure that each of Ellen's remaining days was full of life—as per her direction.

Two women, two wonderful lives, two very different approaches toward death. Ellen had done important work ahead of time to make sure she would be able to concentrate on what mattered to her most at the end of her life. Liz, arguably, wasn't as well-prepared, and her lack of preparation—what I might call her lack of "death literacy"—caused her and her loved ones distress.

Most of us probably fall somewhere between these two women in what we want and how we wish to prepare, but it is instructive to see these strong women represent either end of the spectrum.

I have this great calendar on my office desk. September's message really resonated with me: "The world is not going to come to you. The sooner you realize this, the more time you'll have to pack." If I were designing a calendar for this chapter it might read instead, "We are all going to die. The sooner you realize this, the better you can prepare for death and get on with living." In this chapter, I will talk about what it means to be literate about death, why it's important, and steps that you and your loved ones can take to increase your death literacy—and, ideally, improve the dying process for yourself and those around you.

Fear

What's the biggest reason so many of us avoid talking about or planning for dying and death? Fear. Simply put, we're scared. Dying and death can bring out a wide variety of concerns and fears. Some of the more common fears include

- ***Fear of physical pain:*** Dying is a natural process, one that we will all go through. We are scared that it will be painful. We can't picture how we will bear it—and so we avoid thinking about it. Today, most physical pain at the end of life can be managed with medication and access to a palliative approach to care.
- ***Fear of psychological suffering:*** For many of us, suffering at the end of life is one of our greatest fears. It's important to recognize that when we talk about suffering, we mean not only physical but also emotional and social pain. We don't want to leave our loved ones behind. We don't want to cause them the grief we know they will experience. For many people, the social and emotional pain that accompanies dying can cause the greatest suffering.
- ***Fear of the unknown:*** Even if we're well-educated about the dying process (and not many of us are), none of us have actually experienced death. It's normal to be scared of the unknown and be fearful of the end of life. Giving voice to these fears and sharing them with others—even if they don't have answers—can help us to feel less isolated.
- ***Fear of losing control:*** This is a big fear for many people. We live in a society that values autonomy,

the ability to make our own decisions and be in control. Dying is a process where we become more reliant on others; in it, we often need let go of control, to say good-bye to plans and dreams, to become more fluid and adaptable to change. We may need people to help us with intimate bodily functions and activities of daily living such as cleaning, feeding ourselves and walking. Many people fear the lack of control and increase in dependence on others that accompanies dying.

- ***Fear of regret:*** Many of us are scared of death because we fear we won't have lived life on our own terms, or to the fullest. We may regret decisions we took and paths we didn't. Tackling that regret while there is still time to accept and to forgive oneself and others allows a more peaceful death.

Denial: Not Just a River in Egypt

When I was first diagnosed with cancer, I blocked out key pieces of my treatment plan. My doctors would explain a procedure, and it was as though they had never spoken: I didn't take in or remember anything they said about timelines, treatment plans or even details about upcoming surgery. In other words, I was in denial.

As it does for so many of us facing a challenging situation, my denial served a purpose. It was a coping mechanism, like a shock absorber, that protected me from the full impact of a painful situation. I was using it because reality at that moment was way too overwhelming. I could only take in so much. Gradually, though, I began to be able to face my new reality. As that happened, I was able to allow in more information. I was grateful that no one rushed me in this process. My husband and health-care providers understood that denial and hope can be a delicate balancing act. They reinforced the information that I needed in order to make decisions, but they didn't push some of the other minute details on me if I didn't immediately need to know them.

Clearly, denial can be useful. It lets us take in information at a rate we can manage. It can allow us to focus on the aspects of illness or dying that we can actually do something about, without worrying about the things beyond our control. Some people say that denial creates space for hope.

But denial is not always a positive coping mechanism. Unchecked, it can hinder our ability to die well or appropriately. Denial can be a problem, for example, if it interferes with a person's ability to make decisions about treatment or care, or inhibits them from having important conversations with those they love. If denial keeps someone from getting a new symptom checked out or treated, the result can be unnecessary pain or a rapid decline in health that could have been avoided.

So, how do you tell the difference between healthy and unhealthy denial? Since denial serves a purpose, it's not always helpful to try to "take away" someone's denial by "forcing them to face the facts." This is my guideline: if the denial is not hurting a person, preventing them from making essential decisions or affecting their relationships with others, then leave it alone for now. It may well be helping them to understand and slowly accept their situation or the dying process. But if denial is not serving a person well, acknowledge that it is part of their coping but encourage them to consider what they might do differently if they were not spending their energy on it. Often in palliative care we talk about "hoping for the best but preparing for the worst," which allows people to continue using their defence mechanism but can move them toward action and planning. For example, gently suggest that you, too, are hopeful, but should things not work out the way they are hoping for, some plans should be put in place so they are ready.

Moving the Conversation Past Fear

Our fears about death can be vast and existential. We have questions for which there are no answers, problems for which there are no easy solutions. In order to begin to move past our fears, we need to open up the conversation to talk about what can reduce them. When I am working with people in palliative care, I always ask about their fears, but the conversation never ends there. I also ask questions like: What reduces fear in your life? What gives you comfort? What might offer you peace of mind as you face the end of your life? What do you think might make a day good for you, even as you are dying? What challenges have you overcome in the past? How can you use the same skills or resources to help face the challenge of dying?

These are difficult questions. But they are important ones. They help us address and solve some of the challenges of suffering. This is a critical part of the process of death literacy.

Becoming Literate about Death

When we think about literacy, most of us think about reading, or math, or maybe emotional or digital skills. More generally, we're talking about the knowledge necessary to navigate a specific topic. Death literacy involves the skills and knowledge required to plan for and support ourselves and others at the end of life.

Why do we need to improve our death literacy? Because knowledge is power: knowing about dying and death will allow us to make informed and empowered decisions at the end of life. It will familiarize us with the systems and processes surrounding death and let us use them more effectively. Being knowledgeable about death allows us to take a more active role in the care that occurs at the end of life, whether for ourselves or a loved one. Becoming death literate, in fact, comes with a whole host of benefits. For example:

- ***Less fear:*** Many of us are scared of the unknown, and death remains one of the most unknowable aspects of life. I have found, however, that when people acknowledge the reality of death and spend time learning about and preparing for it, they're often less afraid of it.

- ***More perspective:*** A healthy respect for death encourages people to embrace life. This acceptance can inspire us to live fully and deeply and to think about the legacy we want to leave. If we accept that life will end, it's easier to focus on the present and to prioritize the things that matter to us and make us happy.

- ***More pleasure:*** People who have been diagnosed with serious illness often say they become more active in their lives and focus on the things that truly matter to them. They strive to spend quality time with those they enjoy, engage in meaningful activities and use their time and energy wisely. In turn, living life fully and mindfully sets the stage for dying well. When we recognize and accept that life and death are intimately connected, we can embrace life more fully and accept the idea of its end with more grace.

- ***More motivation:*** Understanding that death is a part of life challenges us to complete important tasks. We work to have the important conversations, achieve our goals and have the adventures we dream of.

- ***A deeper sense of spirituality or connectedness:*** Considering the end of life challenges us existentially, death brings up some big questions: What was it all for? Is there life after death? What meaning did I find in my life? Whether you're religious or not, contemplating these kinds of questions can help you feel connected with something bigger than yourself. It can serve to deepen your connection with others and the act of living. It also can help navigate the act of dying.

  When a group of people possesses death literacy, it is not unusual for them to advocate for improved care at the end of people's lives. Knowledge, skills, experiences and social change are all pieces of death literacy. Together these components motivate people to change the status quo, to develop society's capacity to care about and acknowledge dying and death as integral parts of life and living.

- ***More peace of mind:*** Many people report feeling more at ease once they've spent some time and energy deciding how they would like to be cared for at the end of life. Making practical arrangements—such as an advance care plan, a will and maybe even funeral arrangements—allows us to maintain the sense of control and autonomy so many of us value. Many people develop peace of mind through working to get their affairs in order. This can be the case even if they do that planning while they still anticipate having many decades of healthy life ahead.

So, how do we become more death literate? How do we improve the conditions under which we die? How do we increase our access to appropriate and timely health care, medications, professional supports? How do we feel at ease with where we die and our state of mind as we approach death?

Advance Care Planning

In Canada, advance care planning is an important way to improve the odds of dying well and appropriately. In the past, a document that outlined your wishes and preferences for care was called a "living will." In Canada, we now largely refer to this as an "advance care plan." Depending on where you live in Canada, this document may or may not be considered a legally binding document and it may be called a different name, such as a living will or health-care directive. The Canadian Hospice Palliative Care Association describes advance care planning as a process of reflection and communication. It's the opportunity for people to consider their values and wishes and to let those accompanying them throughout their dying process know what is important to them.

Advance care planning helps people to maintain some control over how they are cared for, the kind of treatment they receive, where they die and who accompanies them through the dying process.

Advance care planning is not a one-time event. Rather, it is an ongoing process that that may change over time. It is crucial that we talk with those who love us about our hopes and fears, and with our health-care providers as we discuss the realities of our diagnosis and health status so that they are aware of our choices. We need to think of what we want for ourselves, but sometimes we will need to encourage a loved one to think about an advance care plan for them as well.

The following questions can help you and your loved ones begin to think about advance care planning:

- What might your future health challenges be?
- What kind of care do you think you might want or need? If you are ill or in pain, how can your symptoms be controlled and your death be peaceful? What are your thoughts on balancing pain versus alertness?
- Ideally, where would you like to die?
- What do you think will be important to you at the end of your life—for example, seeing your grandchildren, being at home as long as possible, being able to be independent, minimal pain?
- Are you afraid of death? Why or why not? What are your fears around death? What might help alleviate those fears?

- Do you have any unfinished business that you need to address before you die? What is it and what steps could you take to resolve it?
- Which people will be important to have around you at the end of your life?
- Who do you trust or want to help provide care for you, or to make decisions for you if you can't make them on your own?
- Whom do you want with you when you die?
- What do you need to do, think about and arrange so that you can die well?
- What plans need to be in place to allow you to die in a way that reflects how you lived your life?

As you begin to think about these questions, write down your answers. A record of one's thoughts, wishes and preferences can serve as future instructions for the people who have to make decisions around your care in the event that you are unable to make them yourself. And the converse is true as well. If your loved ones have laid out their preferences, it will be easier for you to know the right thing to do.

Undertaking this kind of planning in no way signals giving up the hope of living a long and healthy life. I believe the opposite is true. It does, however, recognize that at some point we all die. Preparation ensures that at the end of our lives we have the dignity, control and choices that we want. Thinking about dying and death allows us to shift our focus and hopes to living the rest of our lives as well as possible.

Substitute Decision-Makers or Proxies

A person who makes decisions on someone else's behalf is called a "substitute decision-maker" or "proxy," depending on where you live in Canada. (For more information on terminology, see the Resources section.) Either way, this is the person who has agreed to be your voice, the person you trust to represent your best interests at the end of your life. Your health-care team will look to this person to help make decisions and guide your care. That's why it's important that your substitute decision-maker understand and appreciate what is important to you. This person needs to be willing and able to speak up for you and to represent your preferences if and when you can't speak up for yourself. Some questions for you to consider when choosing a substitute decision-maker:

- Will this individual listen to and respect what is important to me?
- Will they be able to advocate on my behalf?
- If they see life and death differently than I do, will they still be able to do what I've asked them to?

Dying to Know

No matter how many of us would prefer to live in denial about dying and death, the reality is that death is one of the few things any of us can truly count on. And while death and dying come with many unknowns, we can still do a great deal to prepare ourselves for them intellectually, emotionally, financially and even physically. With assistance from her family and the team on the hospice unit, Liz was able to improve her death literacy and do some of the work she needed to do in preparation for her death. She acknowledged that it was tough work as she was dying and she wished she'd known to do it earlier. Still, having the conversations helped alleviate some of her fears. Increasing our death literacy helps move death from the peripheries of our consciousness to a place of consideration and respect. The conversations, planning and experiences help make death personal, real and meaningful.

CHAPTER THREE

Dying Matters to Our Families

"I don't think you should think daily on it, but I do think it's worth having in the back of your mind, in terms of the kinds of conversations you want to have with your family ... so that they have a sense that you are not there forever."
—Cory Taylor, author of *Dying: A Memoir*

I wasn't particularly surprised when my dad told me and my younger brother that our maternal grandfather—my Opa—had died. I was 10 at the time. I knew that Opa had been very sick, and I thought that he was pretty old, so his death made sense to me, even if it made me sad.

What *did* surprise me was the festive scene that greeted us when we arrived at my Opa's home following his death. We walked through the door to a full house, with laughter, loud voices, glasses clinking. It sounded like a party, the kind of party I'd seen my grandfather throw many times before. I looked at my dad, scared. "Didn't anyone tell them that Opa died?" I asked.

Until then, my knowledge of death had been limited to the movies. I knew enough to know that people were usually very sad and cried a lot when someone they loved died. But no one had ever talked to me about the wide range of emotions people actually feel. No one had told me about the power of reminiscing. It had never occurred to me that it was possible to celebrate a life well-lived with equal parts happy memories and sadness. My grandfather's death, and the ensuing celebration of his life, sparked a turning point in my personal death education. And they were, in retrospect, the beginnings of my understanding that death is very much a family event.

Dying does not occur in a vacuum. It has an impact on the entire family. The field of palliative care recognizes this, often referring to the "family system" as the client or the "family unit of care." Our family is often our first educator about dying and death. We hear stories about family members who have died. We learn from watching older family members as they grieve. We get our direction about how we should act, what we should say and even if we should be scared about dying and death. Often, family is a major source of love, support and comfort during and following the dying process. And just as often, families facing their stress and grief find themselves challenged by entrenched, ineffective or unhealthy patterns of communication. As one family drily told me when the matriarch of their family was dying, "Families put the *fun* into dysfunction."

It is important to note here that there are many different definitions of what a family is, and that "family" means different things to different people. Family members may be related by blood, marriage, experience or any other connection. For the purposes of this book, the family unit can be defined as *whomever the person who is dying identifies it to be.*

This chapter will unpack the communication needs of families during this challenging time and offer some context around how they try to manage, talk to and cope with one another.

We Are Family!

Each family is unique. And because of this, there is no way to predict how a family unit will respond to the dying and death of one of its members. Although many people experience similar feelings when faced with death, they may move through the emotional pathways at different times. Learning that a family member is dying is a painful blow. Especially if the onset of an illness is sudden or unexpected, most family members will initially feel shock and numbness. As time goes on, the information settles in and the knowledge and its effects become part of day-to-day life. Similarly, many family members first try to make rational sense of the dying process. As time passes, their understanding of death moves from the head to the heart and they begin to absorb the larger emotional impact. The speed at which this takes place can be different for each member of a family—and it can cause friction. Families often struggle when members understand and adapt to death and dying at different speeds.

While each family will have different timelines, hopes, requests and ways of coping, in my work I've seen a few commonalities among families facing the death of one of their members.

> ***Families need to adjust to changing roles.*** I remember working with a family of five brothers. They'd lost their parents as teens and now were spread across the country, most with families of their own. The second-youngest of the five—the one his brothers described as the "black sheep" of the clan—was dying. Throughout their lives, he'd been notorious for getting into the kind of trouble that required the other brothers to join forces, get back in touch and figure out how to get him out of the latest situation he had gotten himself into. As this brother lay dying, the others kept vigil, sharing stories of crazy (mis)adventures and mishaps. What, they wondered, would be their excuse to connect once the "black sheep" was no longer around to get himself into trouble?
>
> We all have roles in our family: the black sheep, the rebel, the peacemaker, the social convener, the baby, the "responsible one." When a family member is diagnosed with a terminal illness, those roles often need to change. And when a family

member dies, the remaining members need to figure out a way to continue without that person performing his or her role. For example, if the primary wage earner is dying, other family members may need to contribute financially in ways that they hadn't before. If the peacemaker in the family is dying, the family unit may need to find new ways to connect and interact without that person acting as the intermediary. If Grandma was the family's binding connection before she became ill, her family may now feel confused and disjointed because she was the family member everyone relied on to keep the unit strong and cohesive.

Sometimes, the roles themselves can be unhealthy: the "baby" of the family may never learn to take care of his own needs and obligations. Someone whose role has always been to take care of other people, or to remain strong and stoic, may not give herself the space she needs to grieve or take care of herself—or to allow others to care for her. Family members need to be able to both take care of themselves and support one another.

While some families adapt naturally to these kinds of role transitions, others struggle. Sometimes a different family member moves into the role—for example, taking over hosting a holiday dinner or becoming the new peacemaker. Sometimes, if a person's role in the family dynamic was toxic or stressful, it can be a relief to no longer have to cope with their part in the drama. Still, shifts in roles, both positive and negative, can be unsettling and bring up old or strong emotions.

Families need to care for their caregivers. During the progression of terminal illness, there's usually a time when some family members will act as caregivers. Caregiving may be hands-on as someone provides physical support in the form of feeding, bathing, dressing or giving medications. It might involve practical support, such as providing transportation to medical appointments, cleaning the house or raking the leaves. It can involve emotional and even financial support. Caregiving is not an easy task, and often caregivers report feeling isolated, stretched and overburdened. In Canada, we expect a great deal from our informal caregivers and are just beginning to appreciate the challenges they face attending to their loved ones near the end of life.

Many family members who have cared for a loved one who is dying report that the experience is rewarding and fulfilling. They also acknowledge that it is challenging and exhausting on many levels: emotionally, physically, spiritually, socially and financially. For all these reasons, it's important to remember that those who are the most active caregivers also need support and assistance from the family unit so that they can continue to care for the dying person. Support for caregivers may be practical (such as meal preparation or transportation), or emotional (for example, listening and providing rest time and opportunities to vent emotion).

This can be easier said than done. Not all families participate in caregiving and support the same way when one of their members is dying. Sometimes the responsibilities are shared—and often they are not. Some people are closer geographically or emotionally, or are better in stressful or emotional situations, than others. It's true that some families rise to the occasion and to caregiving challenges almost seamlessly, appearing to know intuitively how to support one another as they care for the family member who is dying. More often, however, disagreements arise: over the right course of action, who's not doing enough, who should be doing what, and whose job it is. In addition, intense emotions, old familial habits and entrenched patterns of coping all add to the challenges of caregiving. As Canadians become more aware of these challenges, support groups or volunteer organizations are forming to offer respite for caregivers so they can get a break. The Compassionate Care Benefit offered by the federal government is designed to relieve caregivers from the stress of trying to continue working while actively providing care for someone who is dying.

Families need open communication. Take a moment and think how your family communicates. Who generally takes the lead? Who usually knows the information first? Who is often the last to know? Whom do you count on for the most trustworthy account, and whose stories tend to need some verification?

Communication is always important to how families function, and it's even more important when a family member is dying, for poor communication tends to be at the heart of much family conflict. For example, some families may try to protect one another by avoiding frank and difficult conversations about dying and death. Some members may believe that talking about death will make it come faster. Or they think that these kinds of conversations are simply too difficult for certain family members to handle.

In fact, difficult conversations often make things easier. While none of us enjoys conversations about death and dying, research done on advance care planning shows that having them reduces feelings of isolation and loneliness. Believe it or not, sometimes it takes more emotional energy not to say what you wish you could say. Giving ourselves permission to express our feelings and concerns frees up energy for more important activities, such as caregiving. It also facilitates necessary connections between family members.

It's important that families find an effective and easy way to share information among all members. If your family is having difficulty talking about the dying process, a good strategy can be to have a meeting with health-care providers. It's often easier for family members to hear and absorb information directly from a member of the health-care team. They can ask questions and learn about what might come next. Many families report that these meetings are beneficial. A family I know used another strategy: they created a Google doc, accessible to the whole family, where they stored and shared information about their relative's disease and its progression and prognosis. Family members involved in doctor's appointments and caregiving updated the document daily. With this kind of strategy, no one can complain that they've been left out of the loop. I will come back to this later in the book and list some good social media platforms that can help families share information with each other and wider circles.

Families need to make decisions. With death and dying comes decision-making. People need to make decisions about treatment: whether to be treated at all and how, and then, if and when to stop. People need to decide whether to take pain medication, when to call a health-care provider for advice or more support, whether to go into hospice care or be treated at home, and so on.

Wherever possible, the family member who is dying should make decisions about her own care for as long as she can or chooses to. It's not unusual, though, for people who are dying to ask their loved ones for input and help to make decisions. Our health-care system tends to prefer it when one person becomes the family delegate responsible for decision-making on behalf of the person who is ill. In many families, it is common for additional family members, perhaps all of them, to want to be included in some important care and treatment decisions. But it is important that health-care providers get unified and clear direction from the family through a point person. You can imagine the distress and chaos created when health-care providers get conflicting instructions from various loved ones.

Sometimes family members, in their desire to help, are tempted to jump in and tell their dying loved ones what they should do. Unsurprisingly, their advice isn't always well received. Being told what to do can backfire, leading to resistance and the deferral of important and difficult decisions. If you're concerned about a decision that needs to be made, a good strategy is to lead with a statement about your concern. For example: "I bet that this is so very hard. I know this is not what you ever thought you'd be doing at this point in your life. I see you trying to make things work but I worry that..." Or, "You probably never imagined yourself having to make these kinds of decisions, but unfortunately this decision needs to be made now. What are your thoughts?"

Death and dying also have a huge financial impact, one we don't often talk about. Dying people and their families will be charged with making decisions about money as well as health care. If the dying person is the breadwinner, what's the impact of the loss of their salary? Do they have disability or other forms of insurance? Who will pay for medications or other care not covered by insurance? What if caregivers need to take time away from work, or hire babysitters? And, of course, what will happen to the dying person's money and belongings after death?

Just as they do with health-care decisions, people may avoid making financial decisions because they aren't ready to accept their deteriorating condition or they have been brought up to avoid discussing finances. It can help to acknowledge discomfort around talking about money, as well as people's desire to maintain a sense of control about their finances. So, a conversation about finances could start like this:

"I wanted to have a conversation with you about money. I know it can be uncomfortable to talk about. And I know you have always been in charge of your own finances and that's important to you. But I'm concerned about what might happen if you can't keep up-to-date with paying the bills and managing things. I want you to know that I'm here to help."

Families need opportunities to say good-bye. I once worked with a very organized, proactive and strong-willed family of three daughters who cared for their mother as she died in hospice. The eldest daughter had a checklist of everything that had to happen before her mother died. Included on that list was saying good-bye. This daughter, it was pretty clear, wanted the sort of heartfelt emotional moment that characterize Hollywood tear-jerkers: cathartic, full of expressions of love and forgiveness.

Mom, however, was not an overtly emotional woman and had not engaged in great displays of affection during her life. She wasn't about to change that just because she was dying—and she told her daughter as much. But the daughter's desire to have this emotional exchange was so important that it began to cause conflict within the family unit, which sided with Mom. "You need to let it go and let Mom be who she is," the younger sisters told the firstborn.

As time progressed, I learned that the mom's favourite song was "Red River Valley." The lyrics in that well-known Canadian classic are all about saying good-bye and the sadness associated with it:

From this valley they say you are going,
We will miss your bright eyes and sweet smile,
For they say you are taking the sunshine
Which has brightened our pathways a while.

[Chorus]
Come and sit by my side if you love me;
Do not hasten to bid me adieu,
But remember the Red River Valley,
And the girl that has loved you so true.

With support from her sisters, the eldest daughter was eventually able to compromise. She exchanged the vision of her deathbed good-bye with sitting by her mother's bedside and softly singing "Red River Valley," over and over. Her sisters joined her. Sometimes, each sang by herself; sometimes they sang with their mom. This was their good-bye.

I had the privilege of attending this funeral. It was a beautiful celebration of life. At its end, the daughters sang "Red River Valley" one last time for their mom. This time, they added an original verse about how much they loved their mother and how grateful they were to have had her in their lives. In this new verse, they had the opportunity to sing their good-byes.

Saying good-bye can take many forms, including songs, letters, heartfelt conversations and videos. Many people find their own rituals. My aunt, for example, also wasn't a fan of big, emotional good-byes. When she was dying, she asked her family and friends to visit her home. There, we found coloured sticky notes and pens: we were instructed to walk around the house and put the sticky notes on the belongings that we wanted for ourselves. We then had to report back to her with what we had claimed. It was important for my aunt to know which items we chose to remember her by.

People need to feel that they have had an opportunity to tell the person who is dying that they are loved and that they will be missed. The person who is dying sometimes also needs to be able to do the same. Often, families need to be reminded that while each member is saying good-bye to the dying loved one, the person who is dying has many good-byes to say. It is hard work and requires courageous emotional effort on the part of the dying person. We need to remember this and to be sensitive to the amount of energy our loved one has left.

Families need to plan after-death rituals like funerals, burials, cremations and wakes, or other celebrations of life. When someone is dying, their family members are often focused on making the most of the time that they have together. The last thing they want to think about is a funeral or memorial service. They may feel uncomfortable planning a funeral while the person is still alive—it may seem disrespectful, or as though they are hastening death.

Still, it's important to have conversations with a dying person about how his or her body will be cared for after death, and how his or her life will be acknowledged and celebrated. These kinds of conversations can provide invaluable knowledge and guidance—it's much easier to plan a funeral or service when you know exactly what your loved one wanted. Sometimes, a person who is dying wants to be actively involved in planning his or her after-death ritual. Other people don't want to think about it at all. Many people will fall somewhere in the middle, providing information about a few key details important to them, and also about what they *don't* want. One woman I worked with, for example, brought up the subject of a funeral with her dying father. Her dad told her that he—like many other Canadians these days—didn't want her to "make a fuss": he didn't want his family to "waste a lot of money" on a big funeral. After all, he was dead. But he did want to be cremated and for his urn to sit in a quiet spot. He let her know that he'd saved some money to cover cremation and funeral expenses and that he wanted to buy a group of his curling buddies one last round.

These were directions his daughter could work with. The family held a small memorial service at a local funeral home. Dad's ashes now sit on the mantel of the fireplace at the family cottage. When curling season rolled around, the daughter cheered on her dad's curling buddies at their first bonspiel and bought the first round. She left the friends toasting her dad and reminiscing about some of his finer games.

As this example shows, Canadian society is moving away from the traditional formal funeral. Still, it's important to have some sort of ritual or celebration to acknowledge the death of someone we love. Such rituals serve important purposes. First, rites like cremation or burial are a way for family members to respectfully complete their care for the physical body of their loved one. Rituals also allow us to acknowledge, pay tribute to and express love and respect for the person who has died. They gather together and galvanize the social communities who will care for and support the remaining family. All of these purposes will be of benefit to family members who are grieving and adjusting to the loss.

It can be hard to begin a conversation about after-death rituals with someone who is dying. One strategy is to position these types of events as a continuation of the kind of care the family has undertaken before death. One family member I supported approached the discussion with her dad by saying:

"Dad, you've told us what's important to you all along since you've been sick. We've tried hard to listen, even though sometimes we didn't always agree. Just as we want to care for you now, we want to care for your body after you die. Can you tell us what you want?"

My aunt was one of those people who plan their funerals down to the last detail. She pre-paid for her funeral, chose her coffin, asked the religious official she liked best to facilitate, picked the music and had my brother, husband and me each audition for the readings she had chosen. But perhaps the most unusual part of her preparation was her insistence that my brother find and purchase as many clown noses as he possibly could before she died. My aunt was a drama teacher who also trained as a clown. She took great satisfaction in picturing all of us at her funeral in clown noses. This unique request added a bit of humour to an otherwise sad occasion. It made us feel good that we could honour her in this way. And no one dared not wear their clown nose.

Navigating Family Conflicts around Death

In a perfect world, when a member of our family is dying, we would all be present, standing around the bed, in perfect harmony. We would be taking care of one another, confident in the knowledge that we had supported our loved one to the best of our abilities. We would be at peace with the fact that we knew and had carried out their wishes exactly as they requested, that communication was always open, caring and frequent, and that everyone in the family felt heard and acknowledged.

Unfortunately, it doesn't usually work that way. Even during the best of times, family members aren't always on the same page. Add the pressure of caring for someone with a terminal illness and of impending death to the mix, and it's likely that even the most harmonious families will experience some conflict. During this very stressful time, new conflicts can arise and old ones can resurface. Family members may have to endure disagreements, bouts of anger, and financial and emotional strain. Many common situations can cause conflicts:

- ***Family roles:*** As mentioned previously in this chapter, different family members have different relationships and roles within the family. Let's face it: we're always going to like and get along better with some family members than others. Every member of a family will have a different kind of relationship with the person who is dying. For some, that relationship will be loving and close. Others may carry longtime grudges, anger or guilt. Past issues of sibling rivalry may surface and bring historical resentments and disputes to the forefront.

- ***Acceptance:*** Family members will accept that the loved one is dying in different ways, if they accept it at all. We all have different experiences of dying and death, and different levels of death literacy. Some family members acknowledge what is happening and take their cues from the person who is dying; others will deny that the person is dying and talk about a cure.
- ***Fears:*** Some family members are comfortable in hospitals and know what the dying process looks like. Others may be scared by the physical decline of their loved one and find it challenging or even impossible to show up or sit bedside.
- ***Distance:*** Many families are geographically dispersed. Those who live far away may feel guilty at not being able to be there, while other family members may resent their absence.
- ***Guilt and anger:*** Similarly, family members more actively involved with the day-to-day caregiving may feel angry or resentful about those who are less involved. They may feel as though they've had to put their own lives on hold, or as though other family members aren't pulling their weight. They

may also feel guilty or frustrated because their care doesn't seem make a difference—the dying person continues to die.

- ***Sharing information:*** Family members may have different access to information. Those in the role of "secret keeper"—privy to information no one else knows—may feel isolated. Those not entrusted with information can feel left out and resentful.

Disagreements don't always mean that there's something wrong or dysfunctional with you or your family—although it certainly may feel that way at times. It's important to recognize that some level of conflict is almost inevitable. In fact, given the stress and change associated with dying and caregiving, it would be surprising if there were none. If you anticipate some struggles in advance, you may be better equipped to deal with them.

Wherever possible, family members can try to be compassionate—with themselves and with one another. Acknowledge the stress. Do your best to recognize that anger and negative emotions may feel personal, but are often about the situation, not you. It can help to look beyond the family: to friends, colleagues, your spiritual community and even health-care providers for support. Some hospitals, cancer centres and hospices have social workers or counsellors available to support families. They can offer counselling to the family as a whole or on an individual basis.

Families are sometimes surprised by their resourcefulness, resilience and ability to care well for each other when someone they love is dying. As one family told me in a care planning meeting, "We've never done the family thing well, but we all love our dad and now Dad needs us, so it's time for us to get our act together." This family managed to put their differences aside and focus on their father. They did this by adopting both a *practical* and a *proactive* approach:

- ***A practical approach*** means asking, "What do we need to make this work?" For this family, it was a binder that kept the medical information and a family calendar that outlined who was responsible for what. They also appreciated family meetings facilitated by a social worker to help them stay on course and keep their goal in mind—caring for their dad.

- ***A proactive approach*** means asking, "When we look back on this time as a family, what needs to happen so we have no regrets?" This family knew it was important to their father that they work together and all be present and involved in his care. None of the family members wanted to be the one who "let Dad down." So, to ensure that they did not have regrets or feel that they had missed out on time with him as he was dying, they focused on the goal of "doing what is best for Dad," and together they cared for him as he died.

Having the Conversation

I've said this before: the conversations that we need to have about dying and death are not easy ones, but they are worthwhile. And they do not have to be sombre or scary events. Nor do they have to be long, formal "occasions," with an agenda that covers all points. Rather, they can be a series of informal conversations that build on each other and provide a gradual picture of what the dying person wants, both during the dying process and after death. Here are some tips and suggestions for conversation starters to help you have these discussions:

> ***Learn from someone else's experience.*** It's often helpful to have a story about someone else so you can put concerns in context. "Did you hear about what happened to Susan's great-aunt? She apparently had a heart attack and died in her sleep. The family was totally surprised as she was so healthy. Her son discovered that she had no will and nobody had any idea about what she wanted for her funeral or memorial service. It turned into a huge family fight. Everyone thought something different and they all wanted it to be their way. That must have been such a challenging time for their family. I'd hate for us to have to go through that. Let's try to avoid that, OK? I'm wondering if it would have been easier if they had thought about..."

Focus on recent news events. As I was writing this book, there was no shortage of tragic celebrity deaths to use as conversation starters. "I can't believe that David Bowie and Alan Rickman died! I hadn't realized they were so ill. I wonder if they had made any plans? Do you think they thought of a substitute decision-maker? I think if I were in their situation I would want that ... How about you?"

Put the "blame" on someone else. "I went to see my physician/lawyer/nurse practitioner/accountant today and they asked if I had made any plans or arrangements in case something happened to me or I got seriously ill. It caught me completely off guard. I realized I hadn't talked with you about what is important to me. Do you ever think about these kinds of things? There are a few things I need you to know about how I'd want to be treated if I got seriously ill, and how I'd like my funeral to go."

Resistance to this kind of discussion is common. I can easily think of 10 other things I'd rather talk about than dying, but few are as important. If the family member you're trying to talk with blows you off, continue to try, gently. Persistence and creativity can pay off.

My mother-in-law is a smart woman who knows an awful lot about many things. Because she's a former nurse, I assumed—incorrectly—that she would have all sorts of ideas about how she wanted to be cared for at the end of her life. One holiday, my husband and I attempted to broach the subject with her. Talk about resistance: she walked right out of the room. Not easily discouraged, my husband and I decided that we would continue to find and create opportunities to talk with her about this. We weren't subtle. When she visited, we placed brochures on advance care planning and palliative care on the pillows of the guest bed. (She has a good sense of humour.) Then one Christmas we gave her Atul Gawande's book on death and dying, *Being Mortal,* and she finally relented. While she still wasn't able to discuss what she wanted at the end of her life, the book served as an impetus for many discussions about what she *didn't* want to happen, which also provided very important information. For example, she knew as a former nurse that if she was diagnosed with a life-limiting illness, she did not want to be resuscitated. She also shared that she never wanted to have a feeding tube. These both proved to be good starting points for our understanding of what she might prioritize at the end of her life. And she also shared the book with her book club!

A non-threatening way to begin the discussion is to say something like:

"Mom, I know you have no intention of dying anytime soon and you know I want you to be around for a very long time. But because I love you and because I want to take care of you just as you cared for me when I needed you, there are some questions I need to ask you..."

Remember:

• Be straightforward in your conversations. Do not mince words or use overly complex or flowery language. Let the person you are talking to know why these discussions are important: because you love them, you want to be able to provide them with the best care possible at the end of their life.

• Point out the possible consequences of not talking now: regret later on, misunderstandings, feelings of guilt and uncertainty.

• Let family members know that what they say today isn't written in stone. They can always change their minds as conditions change.

• Don't give up if your attempts to have a conversation about dying and death are met with resistance. Let your family know that you'll keep trying because you love them and want what's best for all of you.

• Explain your own stake in the conversation: you want to know their wishes so that you can better manage your own stress and sadness in the future.

Many people don't want to talk about dying and death, but even fewer want to be a burden to their families.

No Regrets

I remember working with a woman who was holding vigil as her mother died. "This is only time in my life that I truly regret being an only child," she told me. "Right now, I feel so alone. No one else in the world understands what it means to lose my mother." Just a few doors down, a large group of adult siblings sat around the bed of their mother, who was also dying. Each of them felt a sense of loneliness—because they all had unique and different relationships with their mom.

Everyone dies differently. Every family—and each individual family member—copes differently with death and with grief. This means that the dying trajectory can be unpredictable. There is no road map for the last months or weeks of life for a person with a terminal illness. Families can expect many moments of beauty, but also unexpected bumps in the road. This can leave everyone feeling physically and emotionally drained.

Learning and developing an understanding about dying and death doesn't make it any less hard on our hearts. No family finds death easy. But families can prepare for the challenge. By having the necessary conversations, recognizing each other's differences, maintaining open communication and caring for one another, families can navigate this time so that they do right by one another and look back on these challenging times with strengthened relationships and little regret.

CHAPTER FOUR

Inquiring Minds Want to Know! Talking with Children

"The greatest gift you can give your children is not protection from change, loss, pain or stress, but the confidence and tools to cope and grow with all that life has to offer them."
—Dr. Wendy Harpham, physician and author of *When a Parent Has Cancer*

I remember when my husband's grandfather died. Grandpop, as he was called, had been sick for some time, and his death was not unexpected. Most of his grandchildren were adults, but my brother-in-law's son, Nick, was three years old when Grandpop died. At the time, I did not have a lot of experience working with children or talking to them about dying. I remember wondering how my brother-in-law would handle it.

Grandpop had a full Catholic funeral. The night before there were prayers at which all the family and some friends gathered to say good-bye. Grandpop was dressed in his best suit and was displayed in an open casket. My husband's family is large and enjoys coming together en masse. They share stories and laugh, and this evening was no different. When it began to look like the storytelling would go late into the evening, my brother-in-law decided it was time for him and Nick to head home and go to bed. I remember him saying to Nick, "Go say your good-byes," which was a phrase I had heard him use on a few occasions. Next thing I see is little Nick running toward Grandpop lying in the open casket. The adults, startled by the sudden movement, turned and watched as little Nick pulled a folding chair close to the casket, stood on it and leaned in toward Grandpop. He then planted a big, wet, three-year-old's kiss on Grandpop's cheek and said loudly, "Bye, Grandpop. See ya soon but not too soon." It was a wonderful moment. Nick appeared to understand death in a way that many adults wish they could. My brother-in-law supported his son, answered his questions and then let Nick lead the way. And Nick showed all of us a wonderful way to say good-bye.

Most of us will find ourselves wondering how to talk with children about dying and death at some point. Children will want and need to have conversations about dying and death with the adults who are important to them. Although many children have these conversations with their parents and grandparents, other children turn to adults to whom they are not related for information and support. Sometimes children find it easier to have these conversations with people who are not their parents. They may be teachers, nannies, bus drivers, social workers, coaches, neighbours, doctors, spiritual leaders and other adult friends. Hopefully we will all be lucky enough that a child will trust us to ask us their difficult questions about life and death. Whatever your role with children, the material in this chapter will be helpful.

Children are not usually encouraged to ask questions or talk about dying and death. As one parent of an energetic four-year-old asked me when her mother was dying, "Surely we should give our children a chance to grow up before we talk with them about dying and death?" Most of us try to shield children from pain and sorrow, but dying and death are on the news, in the movies, in popular songs and on television. And it's happening to people they love. At all ages, the subject of dying and death is difficult to avoid.

Developing the confidence and tools to discuss death and dying with children is imperative for parents. Still, it is not something anyone looks forward to. We often feel so uncomfortable that we choose to avoid talking about death with young people. Parents find themselves without support or guidance on how to open these discussions with their children, and they are worried and feel unprepared because no one had these conversations with them. I'm a parent of two and know that my husband and I struggled to talk with our young children about my illness because we did not want them to worry. We thought they might not understand, and we were concerned that we would not be able to answer all of their questions. Like talking with our children about sex, talking about dying and death can be a challenge.

How Young People Are Learning about Death

Introducing children to dying and death does not have to be scary. Nor do death and dying need to be something that we wait until children are "old enough" to discuss. We can introduce death to our young people in a variety of age-appropriate, contextual ways. It's not unusual for young children to be curious about the dead insects and animals they find. They may wish to examine them closely, or they may ask questions about what happens when something or someone dies. Although this interest may seem morbid to us, it is an important opportunity for a child to be able to talk and learn about death. Children should not be made to feel guilty or embarrassed about their curiosity. Their interest may provide a chance for a trusted adult to explain, for the first time, that all living things die and make room for new living things. For many of us, our first experience of death was seeing a dead bird or insect or some kind of roadkill. Research done in the 1990s by George E. Dickinson from the College of Charleston in South Carolina that asked college students about their recollections of their first experience with death found that most involved a family pet. The death of a distant relative or friend, famous people or a family pet is a good opening for these important discussions.

Children often bring up the topic of death in their own time, while playing or watching TV, or when they hear a story on the radio. We need to follow their lead and see where they would like to take the conversation If the subject is raised when we are less emotionally engaged ourselves, it is easier to be clear and candid.

The prevalence of loss and death in children's lives is increasing through exposure to divorce, school violence, media reports of murder and the preponderance of television violence. There is ample opportunity to begin a conversation when a beloved family member's death is not imminent. Take it.

It is also important to remember children are learning about dying and death as much from our inaction as our action. What we choose to leave out and what we share will be what they remember most. As children grow up in society, they learn from it. They absorb its wisdom, its myths and practices, its ambivalence and its anxieties. They can tell how we feel and how open we are to their questions from our verbal and nonverbal reactions. The important adults in a young person's life need to take the lead. They need to open the conversation and demonstrate that it is OK to talk about dying and death. Sometimes adults do not know how much information about or exposure to dying and death a child has had and how accurate that information might be. Without leadership and guidance from a trusted adult, young people will rely on their imagination and experience—gained from TV, movies, books or friends' stories—to fill in the missing details.

Over time, a child will incorporate all the various experiences with and exposure to death and dying that they have had, and their responses and understanding will begin to look like those of the adults in their world. Children develop their ideas about death early, with the most profound realizations occurring between the ages of four and nine. Child development research confirms that most children understand that death is different from life by about three or four years of age. From there, they gradually develop a more mature understanding regarding the irreversibility and non-functionality of death. By nine years old, they possess an understanding of all the components, including personal mortality.

Children, adolescents, young adults and even mature adults are continually considering the social and emotional impact of dying and death on their personal relationships and their understanding of the world around them. What we "know" and understand about dying and death changes within the context of what we know and understand at different points of our lives.

A Child's Understanding of Death by Age

I met grief and death philosopher Thomas Attig at a conference where he was speaking of learning about grief. He shared this quote: "If you are old enough to love, you are old enough to grieve." This is as true for children as it for adults. A child who is less than two years of age will not have a real concept of what death means, but they will still be affected by a death. For example, if a child who is 18 months old experiences the death of a parent, they will not comprehend that the parent has died, but they will understand that he or she is not present and that they miss them. At this age, children will need routine and the active presence of other important adults in their lives who will need to be patient and reassure the child that they will be taken care of and loved.

When children reach three to four years of age, they begin to understand that death means something major has changed in their lives. Often, they do not understand the finality of death and will think that the person who has died has just gone away temporarily and will return. Adults can contribute to this belief when they say things like "Grandma has gone for a long trip." This age group also does not comprehend the inevitability of death and sees it as an accident, something that could be prevented or avoided. My nephew Nick seemed to have an understanding that Grandpop was dead, but he also appeared to think that he would see him again. Although that belief could be attributed to the family's religious belief that we will all meet again in heaven, it can also be explained by his inability to understand the finality of death. Nick's dad needed to explain to him numerous times that Grandpop was not asleep and would not be there for Christmas or other family celebrations. He was not on a long trip, but rather his body did not work anymore and he had died.

By five and six years of age, a young person can grasp many components of a mature concept of death, including the fact that it is final. They understand that when a person has died, they are not coming back to life. Although they may comprehend the permanence of death, they think it only happens to other people, their grandparents, for example, whom they perceive as being old. This age group does not recognize personal mortality and does not understand that they, too, will die one day. They will need the important adults in their life to answer their numerous questions in a way that makes them feel safe.

A child who has reached nine to twelve years of age should have developed a full understanding of all components of death. They recognize that it is final, inevitable and will one day happen to those they love. A child at this age will have challenging questions about the biological processes of dying and might become interested in what happens to the body after death. She may appreciate reading books about dying and may want the opportunity to speak with a health-care provider about what happens when someone dies.

When a person enters their teenage years, they realize that they, too, will die one day. As a defence, or perhaps as a form of defiance, they may act as if they do not care about their mortality and may engage in reckless and dangerous behaviours. Teens will sometimes intellectualize or romanticize death and may try to act as if they are indifferent to the death of someone close in an attempt to protect themselves. Although they may understand the components of death, it will take years for them to develop a deep appreciation for what dying and death mean to them and the role they will ultimately play in their lives. Teens will look for ways to normalize their experience with death and often respond well to peer-support groups. Parents may find it helpful to find another trusted adult who is less of an authority figure to engage the teen in these conversations.

Decoding the Myths

Our society is full of myths and misconceptions about children and their understanding about dying and death that we need to debunk:

- ***The child does not know.*** Children pay close attention to what is happening with the adults they rely on and love. This is one of the ways they learn. They will sense from the adults around them that something has changed. Depending on their age, their imagination may kick in and they may picture a scenario scarier or more harmful than what is actually happening. This is particularly relevant to children at ages three and four, who have active imaginations.

- ***The child is too young.*** Children begin to learn about dying and death from an early age. We need to gear our conversation to their age and maturity, but we must address their questions and curiosity. Teachable moments, such as the death of a bird, can help to facilitate this.
- ***If the child is not talking about it, neither should we.*** Sometimes parents and adults want to protect their children and not make them sad, and children often feel the same way about their elders. Chances are the child is waiting for permission to talk about dying and death and wants to make sure that their parent is willing to talk with them. This is particularly relevant for older children, who are closely observing the adults in their world to learn how they should talk about or act around dying and death.

Children may have lots of questions or just a few. Their questions will primarily revolve around three themes: cause, catch and care. They will want to know if they or anything they did was the cause of the death. At five and six years of age, they tend to be very concerned about their actions getting them in "trouble." Up to ages nine or ten, there is often a worry that they will "catch" whatever it was that caused the person to die. They will want to be reassured that they will be kept safe. And finally, they will have questions about how the death will affect them personally. Children will need reassurance that regardless of who died, they will still be cared for and the adults in their life will be there to support and nurture them.

- ***It is better to say nothing than the wrong thing.*** When we speak with love and respect to young people, it is hard to say the "wrong" thing. Not saying anything communicates something to children as well. When we open the door to conversations about dying and death, we are letting children know that it is OK to talk about this and that we are people with whom they can have these conversations safely.
- ***There will be a "right" time.*** These conversations are never easy or straightforward. There are teachable moments that will arise and it is important to take advantage of these. But sometimes we will not be able to wait for a child's curiosity to start the conversation, and we will have to initiate it.
- ***Children often like to ask big questions at bedtime.*** For some, this is a stalling technique, but for others, they feel safe and secure in their

bed, so they feel that this is a good time for them to ask.

And, of course, there will be children who do not ask questions. They will wait until a trusted adult begins the conversation. Bedtime can also be a good time to initiate these conversations, feeling warm and safe. The trusted adult could say something like "There's a lot going on for you right now. I'm wondering if you have any questions about what is happening?" And if that doesn't initiate anything, try normalizing what you expect the child might be feeling. "When I see your mom so sick, it really makes me sad."

- ***Children should not be at the bedside of someone who is dying.*** Children learn by seeing and doing. We can normalize dying and death by including children in visiting and being at the bedside of loved ones who are dying. They may also be included in gentle caregiving tasks, such as reading aloud or bringing a loved object to keep the person company.

  It's important to prepare the child before they see their dying loved one the first time. Adults need to explain what children will see, hear and smell, how people may behave, and if there are any family or hospice/hospital "rules" that must be respected.

- ***We need to protect the child.*** We are not protecting our children by not having conversations about dying and death with them. We protect them best by giving them honest information in a kind and loving way that allows them to feel safe to ask questions and express emotion.
- ***It is better to wait until death is certain.*** If we wait, it will be too late. We need to take advantage of day-to-day opportunities and teachable moments to initiate discussions about dying and death.
- ***The child will become consumed by death.*** Children will ask lots of questions until they feel that they are beginning to understand. But children are also easily excited and distracted by life and living. They manage to integrate dying and death into life and living much easier and seamlessly than adults do. We have lots to learn from them.

We adults fall into these misconceptions because we want to protect our children. We have an opportunity to make sure that the next generation is more comfortable with death than we were taught to be. If we can do this, then they will be better prepared than most of us have been.

Paying Attention to the Language We Use

Sometimes, despite our best intentions, we flub this talk. One of the ways we get it wrong is with the language we use. Instead of having open and frank conversations, we use euphemisms to cover our own discomfort. This often confuses children and teaches them that the topic is taboo. It is normal for adults to want to protect children, to keep them from the sadness and often difficult times associated with dying and death. But the euphemisms merely obscure what we really need to be talking about, and this is no help to the children who sense that you are hiding something.

Think for a moment about some euphemisms you might have used to describe death, maybe even words your own parents used with you—"got called home," "passed on," "no longer with us," "sleeping with God" (or another religious figure), "crossed the rainbow bridge" (in relation to the death of a much-loved furry family member). Perhaps we are trying to cover up our own fear of death by thinking that we are protecting our children from the hardest truth of life—that it always ends. We must tackle our own reluctance to talk about death. We owe it to the children in our lives to explain dying and death in a way that is clear and honest. Until kids approach adolescence, they are concrete, black-and-white thinkers and they need us to be straightforward with them, even if this feels callous or harsh to us.

Here are some common words and phrases that are often used to distance us from the harsh reality of dying and death. We know how to read the subtext of these euphemisms but children are just confused by them:

- ***"Passed away."*** This phrase is the most common substitute for the word "died." It is used in a variety of contexts, including at school and in church, and most adults understand its meaning. Children, however, generally do not.
- ***"She's in a better place."*** For well-meaning adults who use this phrase, it usually means that the speaker believes the individual is in heaven or some other form of afterlife. The phrase is meant to suggest that the individual who has died is no longer in pain or suffering. To children, however, this means they went somewhere really cool. And who doesn't want to go somewhere cool and "better"? Even children who understand the concept of heaven and an afterlife might not be able to imagine or comprehend a place better than what they are experiencing here on Earth with their family, friends and toys.
- ***"He's just sleeping,"*** or ***"He went to sleep forever."*** Some children have enough challenges with sleep as it is. They do not need well-meaning adults to tell them that a person who has died is

just sleeping. Children go to sleep at night expecting to wake up in the morning and continue living. If we tell a child a dead person is sleeping, we run the risk of them believing the dead person will wake up, or of making them terrified of falling asleep themselves in case they might not wake up.

- ***"She went away."*** It is important that we do not tell a child that the person they love who died in fact just went away. This can lead to feelings of abandonment, guilt about making their loved one leave, confusion/concern about why the person left and/or hope that they will eventually return. Regardless of their response to this well-intentioned statement, the child will end up confused and uncertain about what they might have done to make their loved one go away and wonder when they will return.

Sam

This story about a dynamic and energetic young boy illustrates the importance of our choice of words when talking with young children about dying and death.

I had the privilege of supporting six-year-old Sam, who was in Grade 1 the year his mother was dying of cancer. Sam's mom had a aggressive form of breast cancer, and she and his dad tried hard to take care of him as well as they could while his mom was dying. Instead of saying "dying" to Sam, they explained to him that his mama was "passing." They thought this was gentler and less scary-sounding. Sam's beloved mom died in the late winter. Mid-spring rolled around and Sam's father called me. Sam was acting out and hitting at school, yelling at home, not sleeping well—all stuff that was out of the ordinary for him. Sam's dad brought him to my office. Sam remembered me clearly. He climbed onto my lap and we started to chat. And guess what? This little guy was scared. Everyone at Sam's school was talking about the end of the school year and talking about "passing." He did not know what passing at school meant but he did know that his mom had passed—and she never came back.

It pains me to this day that I allowed Sam to get so confused. Not talking about death didn't protect him; he was still hurt even though we didn't use the "D" words. Instead we confused him and maybe even did more damage. He needed us—his family and his mother's health-care team—to talk about dying and death, to explain to him what those words mean. And the family needed me, as someone who has a lot of experience with dying and death, to support them in using language that would not confuse their young son, to correct the terrible error we had all committed.

How to Explain Dying and Death to a Young Person

Instead of these well-intentioned but confusing phrases, there are kid-friendly ways to approach a conversation about dying and death using clear language and simple explanations. Here are some suggestions:

> ***Cancer:*** You can say that this is an illness or sickness in the body but not the kind you can catch like you do a cold. Depending on the type of cancer and the age of the child, this explanation can be expanded. If the cancer has a tumour, it can be explained as a sickness that causes a lump or a growth in the body that should not be there. A blood cancer may be explained as something wrong with the blood or the insides of the bone.
>
> ***Hospice:*** This is a place where people who are dying go to be cared for by doctors, nurses and other people who know how to keep them safe and comfortable. Sometimes this in a building, a bit like a hospital. Other times hospice care is provided in a person's home.
>
> ***Palliative care:*** This is a special kind of health care provided to people when they are very sick and dying. This kind of care helps to make sure

that the person you love is comfortable and not in pain.

Dead: This means that a body has stopped working and will never work again. The body cannot move, breathe, think, feel, see, smell or talk. The body does not feel pain, hunger or fear. For example, when dogs die, they do not bark or run anymore; dead flowers do not grow or bloom again.

Cremation: This is a process that occurs after a person has died. It is when a dead body is put through very high heat, like in a fire or furnace, causing it to break down into small pieces that look like sand or dirt. Some people choose to do this instead of being buried in a coffin in the ground.

Urn: This is the name given to the special container that holds the ashes of a person's body after the body has been cremated.

Embalming: This is a procedure done at the funeral home to prepare the body to go into the coffin and then be buried.

Funeral home: This is a business that helps a family prepare and arrange to take care of the body of the person who has died. This may include buying a coffin, arranging a funeral and transporting the body. The funeral service is often held in a special room in the funeral home.

Funeral director: This is a person who works at the funeral home and coordinates picking up the dead body from the location where a person has died. This person works with the family to make preparations and care for the body until after it is buried or cremated.

Viewing: This is the time before the funeral when people can come to see the body of the person who has died and share their memories and their love of the person who has died with one another.

Funeral: This is a gathering of people who knew and loved the person who died. It can be at a church, a funeral home, a cemetery or any other location. Often it involves songs, readings, memories and prayers for the person who has died.

Eulogy: This is a special speech given by someone close to the person who died. It tells the story of their life, what made the person special and how they will be remembered by those who knew and loved them.

Hearse: This is the special car that transports the coffin or casket with the dead body to a funeral home and/or to a cemetery.

Burial: A burial occurs after a person has died. It is when a dead body is placed carefully in a special box and then lowered into a hole in the ground. This hole is dug specially to bury the person who has died and is located in a cemetery.

Cemetery: This is a special place where people are buried after they die. There are often lots of trees and green grass around. Tombstones or markers are placed where people are buried with their names and important dates on them so that people who loved the person know where they are buried. Some people like to go and visit where a person is buried because it makes them feel close to the person who has died.

Coffin or casket: These words describe a special box used to bury a dead body in. It is made of wood or metal, with carrying handles and a top that can be opened and closed. The inside looks like a little like a bed with a pillow.

Grave: This is the name for the special hole that has been dug in the ground in the cemetery to hold the coffin or casket. The coffin is buried in the ground and the tombstone marks the place.

Grief: This is the word that is used to describe all the different feelings that occur when someone you care about is dying or has died, such as sad, mad, confused, worried, abandoned, happy or lonely.

As a parent or close family member or friend, you may have this conversation with a child. Or you may ask for the help of a member of the health-care team if you don't feel that you can have this conversation at the time. The person you designate to have this conversation should touch base with you afterward to let you know what was discussed and where the child might be in their thinking about and understanding of about the situation. Here are some suggestions I would make to anyone who needs to have this painful but necessary conversation with a child:

Offer reassurance. Reassure the child that the illness or fact that their loved one is dying is not their fault. This type of irrational thinking happens at many ages and levels of maturity, and a child might need to hear repeatedly that nothing they did caused it and that it has nothing to do with anything they did, said, thought or dreamt about.

Explore fears. Encourage children to name what they are scared of. Ask, "What are you afraid is going to happen?" Depending on the age of the child, this question can show what they are worrying about and what their level of understanding is. Some children may engage in "magical thinking" or bargaining thinking that causes them to believe that if they are really well-behaved or do something extra special, their loved one will be healed. Staying abreast of a child's concerns, fears and confusions allows the adult to gain insight into the child's worries and burdens so that they might then be able to help them.

Provide information. Keep children informed in an age-appropriate way. Children need information to help them prepare for what is happening in their world. For example, a child might need to hear that Mommy will need to sleep at the hospital to take care of Grandma for a few nights. Or that Dad is unable to walk by himself anymore, but the child could push him in the wheelchair. Or Grandpa is getting medication to help him not have pain, but the medication also makes him sleep a lot.

Cry. Encourage parents to not be scared to cry in front of their children. When adults show emotion, it lets children know that crying is normal when you are sad. We cry when we see someone we love in pain, or sick or dying. We cry because we love them. Our tears are one of the ways we show this.

Stay open for questions. Let your children know that they can ask you questions. Most parents assume that their children know this, and while most children *do* know this, they confide that they don't want to bother their parents with their questions at a difficult time. Keeping the lines of communication open is important.

Get support. Trust and use other adults to have these conversations so that it is spread around a number of grown-ups. It is important for children to learn that they can talk with people other than their parents and ask them questions, too. These adults can be extended family members, spiritual-care advisors, teachers, coaches, friends of the family and, of course, healthcare providers.

Repeat. Always try to convey information slowly to children, recognizing that it takes time for a message to sink in. Having the conversation more than once also signals to the child that it is OK to talk about dying and death, and that it is not a topic we need to avoid. If we adults avoid it, we send a powerful message: "If Mummy and Daddy can't talk about it, it really must be bad, so I better not talk about it either." Talking regularly about a loved one's illness and impending death normalizes the message and provides opportunities for children to open up and share their feelings and thoughts when they are ready.

It's OK not to have all the answers. We need to admit when we do not know the answer to a child's questions, but we also need to promise to work with them to figure out an answer together.

An honest "I just don't know the answer to that one, what do you think?" may be more comforting than an explanation made up on the fly just to have an answer. Children usually sense our doubts, and they sure can ask the tough questions. White lies and misinformation, no matter how well-intended, can create uneasiness and distrust. Our children will learn that we are not all-knowing soon enough. We can make that discovery easier for them if we calmly and matter-of-factly share with them that we do not have all the answers. Like them, we are learning from life. This accepting attitude toward having questions for which we do not have answers may also serve to help children feel better about not knowing everything either.

Include children. Children do not like to be left out. Include children whenever possible in visiting, planning and even basic caregiving to show them that it is important to take care of people when they are sick and dying. Children may develop unnecessary fears if they are left out and become anxious when they are not certain what is going on.

Talking to My Own Children About My Cancer

Regardless of how kid-friendly we make our language, having conversations about dying and death with children is challenging, despite the experience we might have. Talking to children about dying and death was one of my favourite parts of my job on the hospice unit, but I developed a whole new appreciation for it and how challenging it can truly be for parents when I was diagnosed with cancer and had to talk about it with my own children. I would like to share my own personal experience. I call this tale "Mommy has a tumour; now, let's go buy a trampoline!"

In my defence, we'd been talking about getting a trampoline before I was diagnosed with colon cancer. My husband and I thought it would be a good addition to our collection of outdoor playthings. Yes, we knew the risks, but working in palliative care, we've always tried to live knowing you could be hit by a bus any day. Six years ago, I felt like that bus had actually decided to take aim.

One of the first things friends asked upon learning that I was diagnosed with cancer was "What have you told your kids?" Talking with children about illness, death and dying was something I used to consider myself good at. It was part of my job as a social worker on a hospice unit. I used to wonder why people found it hard to talk with children. I often found it easier to talk with children about the tough stuff of life than the adults.

Then I had my own children. And when I was diagnosed with cancer, it suddenly wasn't so easy or straightforward. It's hard to talk with your children when the soundtrack playing in your head is "How could you do this to them?" and your heart feels like it just might actually break.

The simple answer to the question "What have you told your kids?" is "We tell them everything we know." Here's what happened.

We called a family meeting on a Saturday afternoon, about 36 hours after I got my diagnosis. Before we could tell our son and daughter, my husband and I needed some time to sit with the information and try to make sense of things. We needed to find something tangible for us all to hold on to. In my family's case, this was a plan of action. So, when my husband and I were ready, the four of us sat on the couch, cuddling under a blanket. We talked about how I'd been sick lately and was very tired. Then we told our children that the test that I'd had a few days earlier showed I had a tumour growing in my colon. I would need to have an operation to cut it out. This operation had to be done in Toronto because there was a very special doctor there who could help me. Then we told them the plan was to go to Toronto as a family. We'd have some fun, and then Granny would take them home on the plane before my surgery. Their response was to run upstairs and pack. They are definitely not ones to miss out on an adventure!

My son, who was five at the time, initially responded by becoming a bit more cuddly and affectionate. He didn't really say much, he just wanted lots of hugs.

My daughter, then aged six and an "old soul," was a different story. Almost every night when we were doing our "goodnight ritual," she would come up with a new question. I knew to expect the big one: "Mommy are you going to die?" Nonetheless, it was still hard when it came. I refused to lie to my children, but I also didn't want them to know that their parents were scared shitless (pun intended). So I told her, "We have a plan that we feel good about. Should it ever change and I don't feel good about the plan, I'll let you know that, too." The plan was the "tangible piece" my husband and I needed to be able to give to our children. We knew that their little worlds were going to be rocked. But we also needed them to know we had a plan for all of us to regain our footing, at some point.

After the "Are you going to die?" question, next was "Can you catch cancer, like a cold?" That was much easier. We never discussed genetics or our familial history of the disease (my paternal aunt died of colon cancer when I was pregnant with my daughter), and how that might increase the possibility of one of them eventually getting colon cancer, too. Both my husband and I felt they were just too young for all that technical mumbo jumbo. And to be honest, I worry about that enough for all of us.

I remember taking my children to see a horse show. Both my daughter and I love horses. About 45 minutes into the show, the three of us were having a good time, munching on some treats, when my son piped up, "You know, Mama, if you were to die, I'd be pretty sad. I probably wouldn't get out of bed all day." To which my daughter joined in, "If you died, I'd be really quiet at school. I wouldn't feel much like talking or organizing my friends." I couldn't say anything other than "Thank you." I hugged both of them and thought, "If I die, I'm going to feel cheated out of time with the two of you."

This brings me back to the trampoline. It sat right outside the kitchen window so that I could watch my children jump. It allowed me to have some space, time to talk on the phone, email, think and cry.

I've learned a lot from my children. Young people don't generally spend a lot of time in intense emotion. They take a more "ebb-and-flow" approach. We adults could take a hint from that philosophy. I still, and probably always will, appreciate a good wallow. Sometimes I like to sit in my wallow for a really long time. My children have taught me that there is space for sadness. But right around the corner, there will be something good, and you've got to be ready to enjoy it. Life is messy and dynamic, and sometimes you just need to go out and get a trampoline.

Like most things in parenting, talking with children about dying and death is not easy, and for us it was easier to do before we were parents ourselves. But the hard work will pay off. Take a moment and think back to how you learned about death. Now think about how you would like this experience to be for your child. Think about how you might approach making this a better experience for your children, and how your family makes space for death in the middle of life and living. Hopefully you will not need a trampoline to do it.

Talking to Other People's Children

While I was a social worker on a hospice unit, it was often my role to talk to children about dying and death. I felt very honoured when a young person would trust me with their questions and fears. As an outsider to the family, I understood that my role was an important one. It's often easier and sometimes less scary for a young person to ask their questions of an adult not closely associated with the person who is dying. The young person might worry less about making that adult cry and therefore be willing to speak more openly.

Some parents and other adults had been very open with the children in their midst, while others had not specifically communicated anything and were not exactly sure what the young people knew or understood. So, once I had broken the ice with a child, one of the first questions I would ask would be something like "Why is your mom/dad/loved one here?" Or, "What do you think is going on with your mom/dad/loved one?" Open-ended questions are open invitations to talk, share and explain.

Before I spoke with a young person, I would make sure I had permission to do so. More often than not, the family was grateful and almost anxious for someone to talk with their child and see how they were. Sometimes parents would say, "We do not want you to tell Emily that her grandmother is dying. We don't want her to get too sad and give up hope." It is the right of the family to put some limits on discussions outsiders have with their children. When a family member would share a variation of this statement, I would first reassure them that I understood that they wanted to protect their child, and that I appreciated that they were concerned about their well-being. I would let the parents know I would do my best to respect their requested limits on my conversation with their child, but I would not lie. And I'm sure you know this next part. Children are not stupid. They are always watching, observing and working to understand the world around them. They know when their parents are scared and are not sure what to say to them. They see them trying not to cry and pretending that everything is normal. Sometimes a young person is searching for someone they can talk with who will not be upset by their questions. This is when having access to an adult from outside the immediate family circle is a positive contribution. Most times, it was never an issue when a family asked me not to tell a child that their loved one was dying. I did not have to. The child already knew this in their own way. They wanted to have someone help them to work through their questions and help them to understand what was going on. I loved that part of my job. It is rewarding to be able to offer straightforward information to help a young person understand what is going on around them.

The research shows that children's levels of anxiety are directly related to whether they are told about illness, dying and death and to the quality of the communication they have about this with their families. It confirms that when children are not given accurate information, they will create information to complete the story. We must not isolate children from death in our attempts to protect them. We need to figure out what they know and what they might be fearful of.

If you are concerned about discussing death with the children in your life, then you are not alone. I found it challenging to talk about my illness with my own children, and I had professional experience and knowledge. But the time and energy were worth it. Death is an inescapable fact of life. We must deal with it, and so must our children. In order to help them, we must let them know that it is OK to talk about it.

This is an important gift that we can give children—our openness and willingness to talk about dying and death and to support them in learning about it. This requires us to examine our own feelings and beliefs so that we can talk to them as naturally as possible when the opportunities arise. Although it can be helpful to know that children may think about death in different ways depending on their age, it is important to remember that, as in all growth processes, children develop at individual rates. It is equally important to keep in mind that all children will experience and think about death uniquely. Each child will possess their own way of expressing and handling feelings. But no matter how they might do this, children need compassionate and nonjudgmental responses from adults as they learn about dying and death. Careful listening and watching are important so that you can see how to respond appropriately to the children's needs. Do not fret too much if you say something that initially feels wrong. You will not damage the child. Mistakes made with love are fixable. Learning about dying and death takes time, and many of us are still ourselves working to understand the ramifications of death and its emotional implications. Give the children in your life a gift: be open to talking about dying and death with them.

CHAPTER FIVE

Creating a Compassionate Workplace

"A compassionate workplace recognizes that the natural cycles of sickness and health, birth and death, love and loss occur within the orbits of their institutions and regular activities every day."
—Compassionate Communities, U.K.

When he was a teenager, my friend Derrick decided that he wanted to work for a certain organization and set about doing everything he could to convince the company to hire him. It did. He started off part-time, sweeping the floors and collecting the garbage. Slowly he worked his way up to positions of greater responsibility and authority. Derrick's co-workers called him "Mr. Safety." His homemade lunches were legendary. He was a dependable and hardworking employee. He was always one of the first to offer help when a fellow worker was having a difficult time or needed some support. Derrick was the go-to guy when you needed an ear, a good meal or help with fixing something in your home.

When Derrick was diagnosed with cancer, his workplace was shocked. When he was well enough to have visitors, his hospital room was constantly filled with his colleagues, who dropped by to keep him up to speed on everything going on at work. When Derrick needed to travel to another city for treatment, his employer bought him an electronic tablet so he could keep in touch. Winter rolled around: when Derrick was too sick to shovel, his co-workers took over, creating a rotating schedule of volunteers who came out at the first sight of snow to clear his driveway and walkways and make sure that he had a clear path to get to the hospital. When Derrick got too sick to climb the stairs to his bedroom, the company arranged for his colleagues to show up one afternoon to help move and set up the pullout bed his wife had bought for the living room.

When Derrick died, his wife asked his employer about the best time to hold his funeral so that his work family could attend. Derrick's company told her to choose the time that worked best for her: they would be there. Derrick's funeral was a standing-room-only event. His company hired another organization to monitor the workplace so that any and all of Derrick's colleagues could attend his funeral and honour their co-worker. Derrick's work family showed up in full force.

In short, Derrick's employer demonstrated how a company can be compassionate and caring to employees as they face the end of life. His company stepped up in a meaningful way when Derrick needed its support. But it wasn't only Derrick the company thought about. In facilitating opportunities for Derrick's co-workers to be there for him through his illness, the company created a positive culture for all its employees.

Many of us spend the majority of our waking hours at work. There we develop important relationships and connections, ones that often extend well beyond 9 to 5. It's not unusual for many of us to spend more time with our colleagues that we do with friends and family, and to develop strong and long-standing friendships and relationships at work. Our co-workers can often feel like our extended family. It becomes more than a job. Just as we take pride in the work we do, we should also take pride in creating a work environment that acknowledges dying, death, loss and bereavement as an expected part of life and living. Then, when we need it, as my friend Derrick did, our workplace will step in with care and compassion.

Think about your own workplace. Chances are, there are already plans in place for life's celebrations: births, weddings, promotions, anniversaries or retirements. Perhaps it's someone's role to get a card signed by everyone, bring in a cake or collect a few dollars for a communal gift. The company will certainly have human resources policies that cover its corporate obligations around promotion, retirement, vacations and parental leave. But what happens when someone is diagnosed with a terminal illness or experiences the death of someone they love? Many workplaces have a scattershot approach to extended illness and death.

They will have short- or long-term disability plans in place for staff illness. They will have bereavement leave for a handful of days for a worker who has had a death in the family. But few will have the coordinated response shown by Derrick's employer.

This chapter addresses three points of view. It is for you to think about the kind of workplace culture you want to have for yourself, should you suffer a serious illness, and ways in which the company can help you get through the death of a loved one, or a well-regarded fellow worker. If you are an employer, it will give you some new ideas about how to build a more compassionate workplace.

It's inevitable that dying, death and bereavement are part of our workplace cultures. When workplaces such as Derrick's create a compassionate environment around illness and death, one that supports employees in caring for one another, those employees will tend to come together in a way that raises the group's commitment to one another and to the organization as a whole. A study conducted in the United Kingdom in 2013 by the National Council for Palliative Care and Dying Matters found that 87 percent of people surveyed agreed that all employers should have a compassionate employment policy, including paid bereavement leave, flexible work arrangements and a range of other support.

Yet many of us toil at workplaces that do not step up in a caring and compassionate way when we need them to. Sadly, too many of us work for organizations that are ill-equipped to handle this responsibility: they can't, won't or don't know how to create the culture of compassion around dying that Derrick's created. This chapter offers some guidance on creating that culture.

Balanced Communication

When an employee is diagnosed with a terminal illness, the employee and employer must make—sometimes individually, sometimes together—a number of decisions about how best to share information about the illness, its prognosis and other details. Discussions about illness, dying and death are challenging at the best of times, and when it comes to the world of work, issues of privacy, finances and job security can further complicate the subject. What's more, we're expected to be "professional" at work and not to become overly emotional or upset. An employee who is ill needs to decide just how much information to share, and with whom. Employers need to balance a sick or dying employee's legal and emotional needs for privacy with the organization's and coworkers' practical and emotional responses to the situation and needs to know more about it.

When an Employee Becomes Seriously Ill

Most people find that the easiest first step when they find out that they have a serious illness is to simply email their boss stating that they have a medical condition that will require them to be off work and that they will follow with medical documentation as it becomes available. As they learn more about their illness and prognosis, they can update their employer with information on things like treatment schedules, anticipated time away or accommodations that may be needed.

Sometimes people will try to hide their illness out of concern that they may lose their job. But employees who become ill while actively employed are entitled take time off work for treatment and recuperation. And a good employer will be both flexible and creative in their attempts to retain the skills, knowledge and talent of an employee who is ill.

It is challenging for the employer to not know how long a worker will be off and in what condition they may return to work, but clear and timely communication can help mitigate some of that. And employers are within their rights to ask for a medical certificate to confirm the illness and that the employee is unable to work.

It is important that an employee keep their employer abreast of their health status, what they are able to do if they are able to return to work, and if there are any medical restrictions that will change their ability to work at their existing job while they are undergoing treatment and during their recovery. If an employee is unable to return to work at all, due to disability or confirmation that their illness is terminal, it is important that the employee inform the employer as soon as they are able.

A compassionate workplace will offer reasonable workload adjustments and recognize that there will be times when the individual is too sick to work, may be hospitalized or need to receive treatment. If the company is large, the human resources department will be helpful about specific job guidelines, sick leave and accommodations. If the company is smaller, a frank conversation with the owner or manager can help both sides make a plan that works for all.

Striking the right balance between these competing needs allows an employer to support both the person who is ill and that person's co-workers, and to facilitate a work environment where people feel both secure that their personal information will be respected and that they have the information they need to function well in the workplace. It encourages the person who is dying to set guidelines about the personal information they're comfortable sharing, and respects those guidelines. It helps that person to maintain a sense of work identity and autonomy during the challenges of illness. It creates conditions where that person's colleagues can share and feel supported in their emotional responses to the situation. And it contributes to an overall environment of compassion in the workplace.

What Makes a Canadian Compassionate Corporation?

The Canadian Hospice Palliative Care Association and its Champion's Council has established criteria indicating that a company has met the standard to be designated a Canadian Compassionate Corporation (CCC). Companies or corporations must meet at least three out of five of the following criteria:

- The company has a human resources (HR) policy that lays out a Compassionate Care Leave Benefit (CCLB) endorsing the job-protected family medical Employment Insurance benefit currently at 26 weeks.
- The employees' jobs are protected while they are off on the CCLB program.
- Compassionate Care leave could provide employees with income top-up of benefits over and above the job-protected family medical employment insurance (EI) benefits leave offered through the provinces and the federal EI program.
- The company has a caregiver accommodation policy that allows for support and flexibility within economic reason.

- The company promotes Advance Care Planning (ACP) using resources and tools at AdvanceCarePlanning.ca or creates their own materials.

Emotional Responses to a Colleague's Terminal Illness

When colleagues learn about the terminal diagnosis of one of their workmates, the reactions can be profound. Responses and their intensity will vary among individuals, and some people will react with shock and sadness and may also experience a decrease in concentration, irritability, anxiety and frustration. Fatigue and mood swings are common. People may feel guilty that they are not doing enough—or feel relief that they didn't get sick. The unsettling news can interfere with an employee's thought processes, concentration and sleep patterns, and all that can have a negative impact on their performance at work. Reduced productivity and increased absenteeism are common. Initially, the responses may be acute and contribute to an emotionally charged workplace.

After a Colleague Has Died

There will be many reminders at first that can trigger grief responses. For example, there will be business or workflow tasks once handled by the person who has died that will need to be reassigned, or a replacement person may need to be hired. This can change the configuration of work groups or teams, and surviving colleagues may feel discomfort or guilt if they move into the vacated space or job role, or they may resent the new hire. A client who has not heard about the death may ask to speak to the colleague who has died. There may be a unique skill or task that the person who died performed particularly well that no one else can replicate at the same level. All these situations can bring up intense emotions.

Every employee will react differently to the news that a close colleague has died, and each will have different needs as they digest the news and manage their sadness. Some will be able to return to routine swiftly and will appreciate the distraction of the work that needs to be done. Others will need more time to adjust before they are thinking clearly again. There are no hard-and-fast rules based on the relationship with the person who died, or the circumstances under which the death occurred, that can predict an individual's response to the death of a colleague or the time it will take for their productivity to return to its normal levels.

Most workplaces, unfortunately, do not have the luxury of providing the required time and space needed for their employees to work on their grief. When it comes to work, life must go on. The job must be done and the company or corporation cannot stop running.

Usually when a family member dies, you are granted a bereavement leave, often a few days. A personal day or two is generally considered the norm when a close friend dies. But when a colleague dies, an entire office cannot stop working, because the company cannot exist without its employees doing their jobs. Still, a compassionate workplace provides an environment that allows people to take care of and be cared for by their colleagues and work family.

Supporting Canadians Who Are Caregivers

As people live longer, more employees find themselves taking care of a loved one with a serious or life-limiting illness. The Canadian Hospice Palliative Care Association (2016) estimates that most Canadians anticipate they would need to commit at least two days per week to care for a loved one who is dying, and that these same people also recognize they will likely struggle to make that required time and energy commitment a reality. Obviously, these caregiving requirements will affect an individual's work life. Employers must be prepared to address this issue, which will often have a direct impact on productivity, performance, absenteeism and the cost of employee benefits.

To assist with some of these caregiving challenges, the government of Canada has implemented compassionate-care benefits for Canadians who are caring for a gravely ill family member. This is an Employment Insurance (EI) benefit available to people who are temporarily caring for a loved one who is expected to die within a six-month period. It offers a maximum of 26 weeks of compassionate-care benefits for eligible workers. These benefits support the idea that Canadians should not have to choose between keeping their job and caring for a loved one. While these benefits are still not enough for many caregivers, they are a step in the right direction that allows people to maintain some financial security during this difficult time. In addition to these federal provisions, some forward-thinking companies also include a paid-leave option for employees caring for a dying family member as a part of their benefit package.

A Safe Place to Grieve

When a colleague dies, members of the workplace will look to management to set the tone for how to respond. It is essential that the workplace acknowledge the death and allow co-workers the time and space to come to terms with the loss of their colleague. An employer that shows compassion and sensitivity will ultimately navigate the grief process more successfully and likely emerge with a stronger workforce as a result. A compassionate employer:

- Sends a strong message to its staff that the organization values its employees—both those who are living and grieving and those who have died;
- Can help decrease employee stress levels, absenteeism and sick leave among employees;
- Ultimately builds increased commitment to the workplace and supports retention.

Here are a few suggestions for workplaces to create a compassionate and caring environment, both immediately after the death of an employee and in the weeks and months that follow:

- Some employees—for example, members of a person's immediate work team, someone's personal assistant or boss, mentor or mentee, or others in a close relationship—will be more affected by the death of their colleague. A compassionate employer will identify these people ahead of time. Wherever possible, they will tell these people first about the death, ideally by telephone or in a face-to-face meeting, and not by email.
- A member of management should then make a formal announcement of the death. If possible, they should call staff together and deliver the information in person. This allows employees to receive consistent information and as a group, and to feel included and supported. This should be followed up with an announcement through the usual work communication channels, such as

inter-office memo or communications bulletin or email. While intimate details of the death don't need to be shared, it's important to acknowledgement the contribution the individual made to the organization.

- If the death occurred in the workplace or was the result of suicide or homicide, it may be appropriate to bring in an outside professional to assist in debriefing the staff. Providing a safe space in which to ask questions and to share information and emotions may be particularly important if the death was unexpected and sudden.
- Many colleagues will want to know when and where the funeral or memorial service will be held, if they can attend, and how they can offer support to the family. The company or organization should ensure that everyone who needs the information receives it, including those who may be on shift work or absent that day.
- As many employees as possible should be permitted to attend the memorial or funeral service with pay. Because this is not always a practical option, it's important for employers to facilitate other opportunities for workers to share memories, acknowledge their feelings and express their condolences. These rituals play an important role in the grief process and help co-workers adapt to their altered workplace now that their colleague has died.

- Decisions about the deceased colleague's job role, responsibilities and workspace need to be handled respectfully and with sensitivity. If possible, these decisions should be deferred until after the funeral or memorial service.
- A close colleague, friend or manager should collect any belongings of the person who has died and return them to the family. Often this is a good opportunity to include a card from colleagues and offers of support. This should occur a few weeks following the funeral or a month or so after the death. Be sure to let the family know in advance that the belongings will be returned so they are expecting this to happen.
- A workplace may want to make a public offer of support or memorial. This acknowledges the death of their colleague and lets the community know that the relationship was meaningful to them. It may take the form of a charitable donation in the individual's name, a gift to the family, flowers at the funeral, a tribute in a newspaper or some other kind of public acknowledgement. Some workplaces have created a memory book or online memorial with contributions from fellow staff who share their stories and memories of working with the person who has died. Management may find it beneficial to involve colleagues who were closest to the person who died in this process. They may have insight into what acknowledgement might be best received by the family.

- It can be beneficial for the employer to create a more enduring workplace appreciation of the employee who has died. This may include a plaque on the wall outlining the person's years of service and the contributions he or she made, or it could be the creation of a work scholarship or award. If the workplace has done something such as this, the family should be informed and be invited to participate if they wish. They could be invited to view the plaque, for example, or to meet the award recipient.
- Management should offer some education about grief and loss and should openly acknowledge the impact death can have on the workplace. This may include some information about the grief experience and where to turn for additional support, such as individual counselling. Some workplaces may wish to implement an employee-assistance program. Any of these suggestions send the message that grief is normal and part of the adjustment to the loss.

Strategies for Supporting Grieving Co-Workers

- Connect with them as soon as possible. Often people feel isolated and lonely in their grief. It may feel awkward to initiate conversation initially, but it is important to acknowledge grief openly. A simple "Please accept my condolences on the death of..." recognizes the loss and may be seen by the person as an invitation to talk more.

- Use the name of the person who has died. Often, we are worried that we will be bringing up difficult memories and be the cause of emotions rising to the forefront. The person who has died is never far from the mind of the person who is grieving. In fact, many worry that their loved one will be forgotten when people do not say their name. Hearing the name spoken acknowledges the individual, the relationship and the loss and communicates that this experience matters.

- If possible, find out when the person who is grieving is returning to work. If it's not you, think of a colleague who is best suited to meeting the person on their return. The workplace friend can welcome them back and again acknowledge the death. Many people who are grieving will talk about the silence they encounter, the elephant in the room, when they return to social situations, including work, and find themselves surrounded by people who do not know how to react to their grief.

- Listen more than talk. Part of the work of grief is to talk about loss in a way that serves to deepen our understanding of it. This process takes time. One of the best gifts colleagues can give an individual who is grieving is an opportunity to tell their story. Do not be surprised if the employee needs to tell the story many times and more frequently during holidays, anniversaries or other special times. It is also normal for tears and sadness to be expressed more freely during these times.

- Do not expect the grief process to be smooth or linear for your colleagues or for there to be a quick recovery in which life returns to normal. A compassionate workplace is one with space for grief, whatever it might look like. The uniqueness of grief is recognized as normal and is accepted. It is still possible to get work done while a person is grieving. There is no timeline on grief.
- If the individual who is grieving appears to be moving into a depression or is exhibiting high-risk coping behaviours, such as excessive drinking or medication use, do not hesitate to encourage the employee to seek professional help. Know what services the employee-assistance program at your workplace offers.
- There will be times throughout the year that are particularly difficult for people who are grieving, such as anniversaries, holidays or birthdays. If possible, try to be aware of these times. Colleagues should not be surprised if they notice increased holiday requests or sick time associated with meaningful dates throughout the year. Grief may actively impact an individual's performance at work for at least the first full year following a death.

While death and grief in the workplace will never be easy things to deal with, the good news is that there are a few strategies, outlined in this chapter, that can be taken to create a workplace environment of compassion and care. Employees feel valued and respected in such a milieu, and this extends to their productivity and loyalty to the organization and the people who work there. A compassionate workplace values employees in sickness and in health, in happy times and grief. It makes space for celebrations of life and death. My friend Derrick was dedicated to his work and created important relationships with his colleagues. In return, his workplace and colleagues stepped up when he needed them to, when he faced the end of his life. These reciprocal relationships resulted in a group of people being committed to making a very difficult time a bit easier through their support and care.

CHAPTER SIX

Navigating Challenging Conversations with Health-Care Providers

"The biggest problem with communication is the illusion that it has taken place."
—George Bernard Shaw

Let's face it: none of us is getting any younger. Not me, not you, and not the Canadian population as a whole. As we age, more of us will develop chronic illnesses, and all of us will die eventually. We need to know how to talk with our health-care providers around end-of-life care. We are becoming more knowledgeable consumers of health care, and we're no longer content to wait for our doctors to bring up the subject of dying. We want to have a say in the kind of care we receive at the end of our lives, and we expect and need our health-care providers to be able to discuss that care with us. Further, we need to have these conversations while we are healthy and able, before the day comes that we can no longer speak for ourselves.

Ironically, many health-care providers are ill-equipped to have these conversations. Some even avoid the conversation at all cost. Palliative care is a relatively new branch of medicine, and an even newer addition to medical education, so practitioners aren't always well-trained to talk about dying and death. In any case, they are usually too busy focusing on keeping us alive to talk to us about dying. That's fine—excellent, actually—when what ails us is fixable. But when our conditions aren't fixable, we need to be able to talk to our doctors about what we want and hope for the end of our lives.

The purpose of this chapter is to provide you with some strategies and communication techniques to best navigate these conversations, which will help both you and your health-care team. I hope they will encourage you to talk with your health-care providers about end-of-life care while you are in the mental and physical shape to have them. Nothing makes illness or dying easy, but open, honest communication can serve to make some things less challenging.

Surprise! It's Hard to Talk about End-of-Life Care

Good communication is essential to good health care. It is integral to people's sense of control and autonomy any time they are ill but especially at the end of life. Research has shown that when patients feel heard and respected and that they are an important member of the team making decisions about their care, they are more engaged in their care and express greater satisfaction with it. And yet, health-care teams often lack good communication skills. Why is communication so challenging for both the person receiving care and those offering it?

Why It's Hard for Patients to Talk

As we discussed in Chapter 2, most of us aren't clear about what's important to us at the end of life. We are uncomfortable talking about death and dying and, when the time comes, we struggle to say what we want.

Aside from our discomfort with the "D" words, communication may be a challenge for other reasons:

- We don't want to pressure our health-care providers or make unnecessary demands of the system.
- We may feel that talking about our hopes, fears and feelings around death is frivolous, an unnecessary luxury. It's a big conversation stopper when you believe that your thoughts and feelings don't have a place, or that talking about them may be taking time away from somebody else's care.
- We're afraid, and our fears prevent us from learning the details about our illness or what may happen next.

- I remember fondly working with a gentleman who readily admitted, "If I don't ask, maybe it won't happen. I'm better off being in the dark." Some people truly do not want to receive information about their illness or prognosis, and this is their right. Every person will navigate this their own way. They may think that they'll have a higher quality of life not knowing, and for a few people, that may be so. Often, though, this form of denial is short-lived. With a bit of probing, we find that knowledge of their condition and prospects is there, even if it not openly acknowledged.
- We're afraid that if we talk about dying, people may give up on us. Or, worse, talking about dying might decrease our will to live.

In the not-so-distant past, people with a terminal diagnosis were told by their health-care providers, "There's no cure for your disease. There's nothing more we can do for you." Today, we know that with good palliative and end-of-life care, we can do a great deal to improve and maximize the quality of a person's remaining time. That's why it's important to recognize that talking about end-of-life worries doesn't mean that we or someone we love is "giving up" on life, or being dark and depressing. Expressing our needs and hopes for care at the end of our lives is all about being informed, about taking or regaining some control by being involved in the decisions about our own care.

Why It's Hard for Health-Care Providers to Talk

OK, maybe it's easy to understand why the average person finds it difficult to talk about death. But doctors, nurses and other healthcare providers confront death every day. Why do they struggle to talk about end-of-life care? It may be less surprising than you think.

- Rarely does anyone go into health care because they want to help people die. Generally, people enter the field because they want to save or improve lives, not help to end them. It's a simple truth, but it explains a lot. I've yet to meet a nurse or physician who said that they entered their profession because it was important to them to care for people at the end of their lives.

- Not finding a cure seems like a failure. Dying is part of living. Too often, though, our health-care providers and systems don't recognize this reality—and this denial doesn't serve us well. As medical care improves and we live longer, our expectations of our health-care systems and providers have changed. Many of us expect our physicians to be able to find a solution to what ails us, and they in turn feel the pressure of this expectation. Cancer treatment, for example, has advanced greatly over the past few decades and many of the cancers that used to kill us quickly are now treatable, with generally high rates of remission. It's not uncommon for oncologists to develop relationships with and care about the people they treat. And no one wants to tell someone they care about that their treatment has failed.

- They lack the education and support to have these conversations. Until the early 1970s, palliative care—let alone training for it—didn't even exist in Canada. It developed out of a recognition that people who were dying from cancer and AIDS were not dying well. They were often in pain, isolated or receiving treatment that was no longer useful.

A surgeon named Dr. Balfour Mount felt particularly challenged by this, and he worked with others to open one of the first hospital-based hospices in Canada, at the Royal Victoria Hospital in Montreal. Like many palliative-care providers today, Dr. Mount did not come to end-of-life care as the first focus of his career. Rather, he identified a need and was called to create change and improve the care of dying people. He, like many palliative-care providers, learned on the job.

Only over the past two decades have palliative and end-of-life care been included in the curricula to train future doctors, nurses and other health-care providers. Even then, they still lack comprehensive training on how to talk with their patients about dying and death. Somehow, we think they'll develop these skills naturally, over time. But that doesn't make sense.

We give health-care providers opportunities to hone and develop other important skills, like surgery. We also need to provide them with opportunities to practise their communication skills.

Good Communication: A Shared Responsibility

The good news is that, slowly but steadily, we're getting better at communicating about death. As patients, we are developing relationships with our doctors and health-care teams that look more like partnerships: all the players contribute to the care plan. Likewise, physicians are realizing that they can provide more comprehensive patient care when they work as part of a health-care team. This may include nurses, pharmacists, social workers, spiritual-care providers, therapists and volunteers, as well as the person receiving the care and his or her family.

Both patients and health-care providers are responsible for good communication. Because communication can break down especially during difficult or stressful times, it's even more important to figure out how to do so effectively when someone is sick or dying. Several straightforward strategies can make the process smoother. Every interaction with your health-care providers is an opportunity to establish or strengthen your expectations for effective communication.

The following tips can help regardless of the setting: office, hospital, clinic, home or via telephone or email. These tips can help if you are the support person for a family member, as well.

- ***Write down—and prioritize—questions:*** Prepare for the appointment by writing down your questions or concerns, as well as what you hope to achieve during the meeting. Your list might include questions about medications, changes you are noticing in your condition or that of your family member or friend, or wondering if something might be done about increased fatigue or a lack of appetite, for example. Prioritize your questions: what's the most important information to cover, and what could possibly wait until your next visit? You may want to share your list with your health-care provider at the beginning of your visit—they may identify items that you can cover together or suggest different priorities, based on new medical information they have received, such as recent test results. You could say, "I have a lot of questions and I'm wondering if I need to prioritize them to make sure we have enough time." This signals to your health-care provider that you respect the demands on their time. It also lets them plan their time with you appropriately.

  Be prepared for the fact that, if you have a lot of questions, they may need to be addressed over a few visits. Your health-care provider can help you plan for these follow-up appointments.

- ***Think about your communication style:*** If you were to receive some challenging news from a health-care provider, what would the best way for them to share it with you? Would you need a loved one with you? Would you like to hear the news but also have something written down? Do you want to have copies of your test results or of medication instructions to refer to later? Would you need some time to think about your questions and to make a follow-up appointment? I tend not to retain information well myself when I'm experiencing stress, as was the case when I first received my cancer diagnosis. So it was always important for me to have someone accompany me to appointments, hear the information, take notes and be able to answer all my questions later. Pay attention to how you take in new information and explain it to your health-care provider. It can help them give you your diagnosis, treatment plan and updates in the way that you're most likely to understand and use it.

- ***Bring a list of your medications—or the bottles themselves:*** It's important for your healthcare providers to know what medications you're taking. Bring a list of all your meds and their doses, or bring the bottles to the appointment. Don't forget to include any natural or complementary health products, such as herbs or vitamins: your health-care providers need to know about them because they can interact with or change the effectiveness of the treatments and medications your team has prescribed.

- ***Keep track of your symptoms:*** Be prepared to talk about your symptoms. Sometimes it's difficult to remember how you feel from one day to the next. It can be helpful to keep a symptom journal. This doesn't need to be a formal document. You can keep track of how you feel at what times in a notebook or on a calendar, or even on your phone.

Answering the following questions about your symptoms can help you communicate more effectively with your healthcare team:

- What symptoms are you experiencing? Which ones are the worst or the most troublesome?
- Are the symptoms constant, or do they come and go? If they come and go, when do you experience them?
- Does anything make the symptoms better? Worse?
- Do any medications help relieve them?
- Do the symptoms affect your daily activities? Which ones? How?

• What do the symptoms mean to you? Can you feel your condition changing? Are you fearful of the changes?

Keep track of your emotional symptoms as well. Physical health and emotional well-being are intimately connected. For example, if you're scared or anxious, you may have difficulty sleeping, which may be reported as fatigue to a health-care provider. If they are unable to address your emotional and spiritual needs, they can refer you to someone who can, such as a social worker, spiritual-care provider or counsellor. Many people find that sometimes it helps to talk about these important subjects even if we know the questions may be unanswerable.

Bring a family member, friend or volunteer to the appointment: Some people find it challenging to attend appointments by themselves. They can be overwhelmed by the amount of information, and worried that they'll not be able to take it all in or that they will forget pieces of it. Many people find it helps to bring someone to an appointment who can support them. That person can be an extra set of ears and can even take notes so that the patient does not have to, especially when the news is challenging. Consider giving the person who accompanies you permission to ask questions—they can help make sure you understand and remember the information.

If you speak a different language than your health-care provider, it's important to bring someone who can act as an interpreter. Family or friends may offer to step in, but it may be a good idea to find someone less connected to you to fulfill the translation role. Doing so helps to ensure that the information is clearly communicated without the bias of someone who may be struggling with some of the news. It also may help you to talk about sensitive subjects or difficult emotions.

Consider a family meeting with doctor: The dying process doesn't occur in a vacuum: it affects the person's loved ones, too. Sharing difficult information can be challenging and painful. Often, people like to receive news and updates from health-care providers, not second-hand through another family member. It takes the information delivery away from family dynamics and into a less charged and more neutral environment. If this is the case, families may request a meeting at which the patient and loved ones can all meet with the members of the health-care team together. It can give everyone a chance to ask questions, talk about their hopes and fears, and develop a deeper understanding of the prognosis and plans for end-of-life care.

Get clear on what you know: Sometimes health-care providers think patients and families know more about the illness than they actually do. Other times, the medical staff are confident that they have clearly communicated information about a medical condition or the progression of a disease—when in fact they haven't. It is their responsibility to make sure the patient and family understand the current state of the illness and its prognosis. It is also important for the patient to talk about their understanding of their illness so that any misconceptions can be quickly corrected by their health-care team.

Sometimes we need to hear the information a number of times before it sinks in and we begin to understand the implications of the news. Many people cope by taking in only small chunks of information at a time, and repetition will allow for this natural defence mechanism.

Ask questions: Don't hesitate to ask questions or to recap what you've just been told. It is critical that you (and your support person, if you have one) understand accurately. If a healthcare provider uses words or medical jargon you're not familiar with, ask them to clarify. It's challenging enough to digest information about your life-limiting illness without having to struggle to understand unfamiliar language. You'll save time and energy for everyone when you ask for clarification. You may want to consider asking your health-care provider to write down any technical terms that are important to know.

If something is changing in your treatment plan, it is a good idea to ask why. For example, you should ask why a physician is prescribing a new medication, ordering a test or referring you to another specialist. And you will want to know what the next steps are. You want to leave your appointment confident that you understand what has been said and what the plan is.

Be honest: As is the case with other relationships, honesty is essential to your relationship with your health-care providers. Sometimes people try to give them the answer or information that they think the providers want to hear. Sometimes people will hide the fact that they are experiencing an increase in pain because they are worried that they might be sent back to the hospital. Or they don't share that they have stopped taking a medication because it makes them too drowsy and they want to be alert. But this is not in a patient's best interest. The healthcare team needs accurate information if it is to give the best treatment. They will be understanding if you want to take a different path, but they need to know. Nor should anyone be ashamed to admit they are scared or confused, or that they don't understand what is being said—this is completely normal, and the team will understand.

No one should feel pressured to make decisions quickly or on their own. If more time is needed to make a decision or digest information, another appointment or visit can be made.

Ask about your options: There are often several different options for dealing with a medical condition, including not treating it at all, or stopping treatment. It can be challenging to make decisions in the face of multiple options.

To best understand your choices, you and your loved ones can ask your health-care team the following questions:

• What are the pros or cons of having this treatment at this time? How might I benefit or what might I lose?

• What might happen if I say no to this particular form of treatment? Might it be offered again as my condition deteriorates?

• What have other people with similar conditions found helpful?

• What should I do or think about now to help me in the future?

Powerful Words and Phrases

As you navigate conversations with many different health-care providers you'll notice that key words surface repeatedly. You'll recognize some, but others will be new to you. Some are medical terms, some are not, but they will assist you in your conversations with your health-care providers.

Hope: This is a powerful word. Sometimes, people are surprised to hear it as they face the end of their lives. But people don't lose hope because they are dying. It's just that hope takes on a different form. When a health-care provider asks, "What do you hope for?" please know that they are not asking if you hope for a cure. They do understand that most people diagnosed with a terminal illness hope for a cure at some point—or even that the diagnosis will be proven wrong. But in this case, your health-care provider isn't doing a reality check to see if you're in denial. Rather, they're asking, "Knowing what you know about your condition, what do you hope for today?"

In palliative care, we speak about hope being on a continuum. Shortly after diagnosis, most hope for a cure. But even if that's not in the cards, there can still be hope. It's just that hope changes its form as disease progresses. Someone in hospital, for example, may hope to visit home one last time before they die. Someone struggling with pain management may hope that they can find a way to make the pain more tolerable. Someone else may hope that the medication they are taking allows them to be alert long enough to have an important visit with a special loved one.

"Do Nothing": Many people worry that if they agree to palliative and end-of-life care, nothing more will be done to help them. That's simply inaccurate. We need to move beyond the idea that palliative care means there's "nothing more" to be done. Certainly, it means that nothing more will be done to unnecessarily prolong the life of someone with a terminal illness. But palliative care is very active. It concentrates on the whole person and their family. It recognizes that a person is more than their disease, and that they have emotional, social and spiritual lives as well. Even if a cure is no longer an option, palliative care focuses on quality of life, on living as well as possible until we die. This active care concentrates on pain and symptom-management, emotional and spiritual support for both the patient and the family and designing a care plan that is aligned with the individual's values and beliefs.

DNR (Do not resuscitate): A DNR is an order, written by your physician, that lets the rest of the health-care team know that, in the event that a person arrests—if their heart stops or they stop breathing—they do not want the team to try to bring them back to life.

There's a lot of confusion around DNRs. Some people worry that if they agree to a DNR they will not receive active care anymore and the health-care team will neglect them. This is not true.

Television shows have done us a great disservice when it comes to understanding how they work. On programs like *Grey's Anatomy,* people are resuscitated all the time. Sadly, TV doctors tend to get much better results than their real-life counterparts. Bringing someone "back to life" can involve cardiopulmonary resuscitation, which may involve cracking some ribs in an attempt to restart the heart. It could involve intubation—sticking a tube down someone's throat and attaching them to a breathing machine called a ventilator. It may involve electric shock or intense medications. It can be painful and aggressive. And if it "succeeds," it may bring someone back to a life in which they are more vulnerable and in more pain than they were before, only to die again from their terminal illness. When presented with the realities of resuscitation, many people decline this option.

Full code/do everything: It's natural for us to want the best care possible for ourselves and those we love. We can't imagine life without them. And so sometimes we intuitively respond to "There's nothing more we can do" with "Do everything possible to keep me or my loved one alive."

But most of us don't know what "doing everything" means. A "full code" means that if someone with a terminal illness stops breathing, or if their heart stops, the health-care team will employ every tool at their disposal to keep that person alive. That could include all the aspects of resuscitation I've described, and could expand to include feeding tubes, transfusions and additional medications.

Sometimes people request "do everything" because they feel that otherwise the health-care team will do nothing. If this is your worry, talk to your health-care provider. You could say, "I understand there's nothing more you can do to cure my disease, but what are you able to do to give me some quality of life now? How can you help me live until I die?"

Advance care planning: Many Canadians are beginning to pay more attention to how they want to be cared for at the end of their lives. Most of us want to have some control and say about what will happen to us, and that is why advance care planning is so important. Earlier we discussed how

> to have advance care planning discussions with your family and friends. Here we will talk about having them with your health-care team. It's important to remember that this process is not just about filling out forms and finding someone to take care of your belongings and money. Rather, it's about having ongoing conversations with those who will play a role in your dying process, and it's never too early to start discussions and provide direction to your family and health-care team about the kind of care you will want.

Just as these discussions are important to have with family and close friends, it's also important to have them with your health-care team. Unfortunately, many of us leave these conversations until a time of crisis, when immediate decision-making is required.

These are not easy conversations to initiate, even with medical professionals. Sometimes people are frustrated by their team's inability to talk beyond immediate treatment options, to address all the things that matter to the patient or those they care for. As a social worker on a hospice unit, I was often charged with reviewing care plans with dying people and their families. One afternoon, I was with a lovely older gentleman who needed to make a difficult treatment decision. Frustrated, he asked me: "How come no one has asked me what *I* want?"

The unfortunate reality is this: if we wait for someone to ask us what we want, we might not get it. Sometimes, health-care providers think they're asking someone what they want by providing them with a list of options to choose from. That's what I was doing with the older gentleman. But that's not the same as asking people directly about their wishes and hopes for the end of life. What's important to them might not be on that list of options, or not offered in a way that is useful.

But by taking these conversations into your own hands, you can turn the available options into things that help you, or your loved one, achieve what you, or they, want in the last days. Maybe it's one last trip to the cottage. Maybe it's to stay alive long enough for someone special to come home. Maybe it's minimal interventions so that your last days are peaceful and blessedly free of any more medical drips and tubes. These are the kinds of wishes that are important to include in an advance care plan.

And it's crucial that you share these wished with your healthcare providers. Sometimes they might need some prompting to start talking about advance care planning. If that's the case, you could begin the conversation by asking a question like this:

"I'm worried about what is going to happen to me if this disease continues to get worse and it looks like I'm not going to get better. What happens then?"

This opener lets your health-care team know that you are ready and willing to begin conversations about what's important to you at the end of life. They should be able to continue the conversation from there.

Some additional questions you might want to ask your health-care team:

• Based on what you've seen with others who have been in a similar situation, what do you think I might want or need as my disease gets worse?

• Will I suffer pain and need medication to manage my symptoms? Will the medication I need be readily available to me? How will it affect me?

• What kind of help and support in addition to medical care is available to me?

• What kind of demands or stresses will be placed on my loved ones? What can I do to help my family?

• What decisions do you think I'm going to have to face as my condition changes?

What Your Health-Care Team Needs to Know about You

Palliative and end-of-life care providers often ask patients, "What do I need to know about you that will allow me to provide you with the best care possible?"

It's a question worth considering. It's worth our while to make sure those caring for us know the kind of person we are and what's most important to us. It will help your team provide the best care possible. What's important will differ among individuals—each of us is unique. When I had surgery for my cancer it was important to me to get home to my children as soon as possible. I also wanted my health-care providers to know that (usually) I had a sense of humour and that was how I liked to interact with people.

But in times of illness and change it's not always easy to filter what's really important to us. So many other worries and concerns are buzzing through our brains. So, it can help to think about what you might tell your health-care team ahead of time. (If you've thought this through in advance, it's easier to remember when you need it later.) I've addressed these questions to you, the reader, but they apply to family members and loved ones, too.

- What is essential that you continue to do to have quality of life? They can be simple things—staying at home as long as possible, hugging grandchildren, taking a shower, walking the dog. Or they can be more substantial—being able to make decisions regarding care, or finally getting married. There is no right or wrong here. It's as simple as what you want and what will give you pleasure and satisfaction.

• What might be your goals for your care? You might wish to live long enough to see an important life event like Christmas or the birth of a grandchild. You may want treatment that will let you stay at home for as long as possible and that allows you to have family close by. You may wish to manage your pain or have secondary infections treated so that in the last days you are as physically comfortable as possible.

• Outside of your illness, are there any extra stresses or major events occurring in your life?

• When you think of what lies ahead, what worries you the most?

• Do you have any unfinished business with those closest to you?

• When your illness worsens, what do you think might still give you quality of life? This might include your relationships, being with a beloved pet, having music surround you or reading.

• You may need to make some difficult choices during your illness and care. Are there any tradeoffs or compromises you'd be prepared to make? Would you be willing, for example, to, be sleepy with less pain, or would you rather be more alert with a bit of pain?

- What does a good day look like for you?

When my husband's grandmother learned from her physician that her cancer was not responding to treatment and that she probably had less than a year to live, she narrowed down what was important to her. She loved playing bridge. So, as long as she was not in too much pain to play, as long as her medication did not make her too sleepy or foggy to concentrate, as long as she was able to brag to her family about her wins, she felt was living well. When this changed, she recognized that she was dying.

Identify your own touchstones, your own passions. What do you love that can continue to give your life purpose? It might be a beloved pastime such as bridge was for my husband's grandmother. It might be being with friends and family. It might be painting, or making music, or writing, or cooking. Think about how you can communicate this to your health-care team, so that they know and understand this about you. It will help them make decisions with you that acknowledge these priorities.

CHAPTER SEVEN

Holding Space for Someone Who Is Dying

"The bitterest tears shed over graves are for words left unsaid and deeds left undone."
—Harriet Beecher Stowe

Many of us are "fixers": we see a problem, we want to fix it, and we search for and take actions to solve it. When someone we love is dying, it has moved beyond our ability to intervene. We can't cure dying. But we are still able to care, and we can put a great deal of thoughtful and meaningful activity into that caring. One of the best ways to consider what that kind of caring might look like is to consider the idea of "holding space."

The phrase "holding space" is getting some good play these days. It may be a familiar concept to people who do yoga or have a meditation practice. On her website, writer and coach Heather Plett describes holding space as "willing to walk alongside another in whatever journey they're on, without judging them, making them feel inadequate, trying to fix them, or trying to impact the outcome." Holding space is a way of offering unconditional support while releasing the need for control. In the palliative-care community, this idea of holding space is echoed in the idea of "companioning" a person who is dying: walking with that person in an environment of care and compassion. Dying can often be an isolating experience, but when we hold space, or companion, we commit to being present and not abandoning our charge when dying becomes difficult.

People have several common fears about dying. These include fear of loss of control, fear of the unknown and fear of being a burden to those they love. Holding space for a person who is dying allows that person to express and share their fears in order to decrease them. It allows people to focus on living until they die.

We can hold space by paying attention to two important elements: the environment and caring communication.

The Environment

Most Canadians say that they would like to die at home, surrounded by familiar things, in a space that they have loved. Yet Statistics Canada notes that almost 70 percent of deaths occur in a hospital. While not everyone who wants to die at home is able to do so, we can do many things to create an environment in which a dying person feels safe and peaceful:

- Bring in some familiar objects such as photographs, or a favourite pillow or blanket. If the person is in a hospital or hospice room with fluorescent lights, consider bringing in a lamp for softer light. Illness and dying can often be accompanied by unpleasant odours, and closed rooms get stale easily. When possible, allow for fresh air to circulate in the room—open a window or use a fan to keep the air moving.
- Sometimes, a dying person may find music pleasant or comforting. If that's the case, bring in some of their favourite music and keep it playing, either in the background or in the foreground for enjoyment or meditation. Music can serve as a means of relaxation and a distraction from pain. It can also be used to block out distracting or irritating hospital sounds. Music is also often attached to memories—it may facilitate conversations and reminiscences.
- It's likely that many people will want to visit when a person is dying. It's important for all visitors—both friends and family members—to respect the person's energy levels and desire for visitors. A large number of visitors can be overwhelming for some, while others prefer it. Honour requests for short visits.
- As much as contact with loved ones is necessary and valuable, a person who is dying may well also need some alone time. This need for solitude can

be particularly hard for loved ones, especially when they know that time is limited.

Caring Communication

Caring communication goes beyond simple conversation. It delves deeper and considers what our actions also communicate. Here are some ways to practise caring communication when someone is dying:

- ***Acknowledge your fears—and then try anyway.*** As I've discussed elsewhere in this book, it's very normal today for people to lack any sort of practical experience of dying and death. Many of us aren't confident that we know how to talk with someone who is feeling lost or fearful. We may not know how to talk with someone who is dying. This lack of experience can leave us feeling lost, worried that we'll do or say the wrong thing and make a difficult situation even harder.

  Don't worry that you don't know what to do at all times and in all scenarios—you can't and you won't. It's normal to feel uncomfortable, scared and at a loss in the face of dying and death. Most of us most will be woefully unprepared and unskilled at dealing with the situation. Try not to add unnecessary pressure on yourself to "do it right." When someone you love is dying, it's OK to be a mess. Be gentle with yourself.

- ***Just be there.*** When my friend Derrick was dying, I would take my 12-year-old son, who loved Derrick deeply, to visit. Before each visit, I'd offer my son some conversation prompts to use. He never used them. Although I wanted him and Derrick to have these deep, meaningful conversations, that wasn't what they needed. The two of them would sit on the couch, like they always did, and just be together. Sometimes they watched TV, other times they ate. On the drive home, I would ask my son how the visit went. "Great," he always replied. "I just needed to put eyes on him for a while." What a gift it is to put eyes on someone for a while and just be there.

  We are a talkative society. We don't "do" silence well. But talking isn't always necessary when a loved one is dying. Often, they turn inward in reflection. Sometimes they or their loved ones will feel things in such deep and complex ways that they are unable to find any words at all. This is when we need to recognize that our simple presence, the act of holding space, lets the person we love know that we care. Non-verbal communication, like holding a hand, a pat on the shoulder or a hug, or your simple presence, conveys your love.

  What's more, dying is hard work: physically, emotionally, spiritually and socially. A person who is dying may sometimes be too tired to talk. In these cases, talking for the sake of filling time and space isn't helpful. So give yourself permission to be quiet sometimes. Just sit together. If you must do something, listen to music, watch TV or read.

- ***Make an effort to be "normal."*** Dying and death are normal life events. While they are challenging, for the most part they are not crises that require our undivided focus. People who are dying know that life continues on, and they often want to be a part of that living. They want to hear about the day-to-day things happening outside in the world. Discuss the news, a favourite TV show or a book you read. Share stories about work, school and family life. Ask the person who is dying to help you work through a challenge at work or help come up with a solution for something that needs fixing at home. We all want to feel needed and a part of life.

- ***Listen.*** Holding space for someone often means doing more listening than talking. Listening can be an important gift to anyone, not just someone who is dying. And yet most of us don't really think about how we listen. We tend to think it's a passive activity that doesn't require much thought or effort. In truth, it's a skill that we should hone. Here are some ways to listen:

  - ***Offer respect.*** None of us understands what the dying truly experience. We need to remember that this is their experience and we are there to respect that and provide a safe space for that experience. While we can share some information, we need not force our perspective or opinions on someone else. We may be tempted to share what worked for someone else, a medication, a treatment or a coping mechanism, as if it will work for everyone. Instead, ask questions about what they think and provide as much opportunity for choice as possible.

• ***Honesty matters.*** It is OK to acknowledge that the situation is difficult, that you don't know what to say or that you're sad. Often in challenging situations we become overly focused on saying the "right" thing. Some of us hide behind humour. While this is very understandable, we do ourselves and our loved ones a disservice by not taking the risk of being honest and open.

• ***Acknowledge the reality of dying.*** Now is not the time to pretend that everything is OK. Do not suggest that things will get better or that the person will regain strength, start eating again or recoup some of the abilities that they may have lost. Avoiding the reality of dying can be a signal to the person who is dying that they can't open up about their anger, fears and sadness. Efforts to reassure the dying person that everything will be OK minimize their feelings, fears and concerns. Instead, hold space that allows them to be fearful, anxious and sad. For the same reasons, avoid platitudes like "Everything happens for a reason," "It's God's will" or "God only gives us what we can handle."

• ***Pay attention to body language.*** Our bodies need to communicate that we are truly ready and willing to listen. Make eye contact. Sit down, put away your phone or magazine and avoid the urge to multi-task.

• ***Focus on breath.*** When you spend time with a person who is dying, listening to that person breathe often becomes a focus. In addition to being a sign of life, breathing can help to slow the mind, make space to listen and help us to stay grounded and calm.

• ***Offer to talk about difficult things.*** Shortly after he was diagnosed, I said to Derrick, "If you ever want to talk about dying, please know I'll do that with you." He looked a bit surprised. He didn't take me up on the offer until a few months later. If you feel comfortable talking about potentially awkward subjects—dying, finances, relationships or sex, for example—put the offer out there. And then accept that the person may or may not want to take you up on it.

• ***Reminisce.*** When my aunt was dying, I visited her in hospice and asked her to let me in on some of the family secrets that I had questions about. She talked about some of her own adventures and spoke of the many people who had been important to her throughout her life. I was familiar with some of this information, but much of it was new. I wanted my aunt to know that her stories, secrets and knowledge mattered to me. Talking about memories can affirm our connections to others and help to ensure that the person will be remembered long after they die.

• ***Be prepared for emotion.*** If you successfully hold space with a person who is dying, you hold space for a wide range of emotions. Emotions are not right or wrong—they just are. Instinctively, when faced with someone's intense or difficult emotions we try to offer comfort. But these emotions need space and time. Try not to rush to the tissue box when tears start to flow. A tissue before it is needed can sometimes communicate that you want the tears to end. Wait a moment. Consider saying something like "You have a lot to cry about —feel free to let some of those tears happen today," as you pass the tissue.

Know that it's normal to cry with the person, and do your best not to feel uncomfortable or embarrassed by tears. Most often your tears won't add more hurt or sadness to the situation but rather will normalize the crying. Tears should be expected when someone we love is dying. They are a natural and human response to distress. Sometimes when we cry, it reinforces for the person who is dying that they matter deeply to us.

• ***Talk even if you don't get a response.*** There may come a point when a dying person is no longer able to respond to you. That doesn't necessarily mean that he or she can't sense your presence or hear your voice. Continue to talk and to include the person in conversations. Share memories and let the person know if someone is visiting. This may feel awkward at times, but it encourages people to maintain a respectful connection with the dying.

• ***Use technology to communicate.*** These days, many of us find ourselves geographically distant from our loved ones. Technology, however, allows us to remain in close contact through email, texts, Skype, telephone or social media. Use these technologies to stay connected through conversations, sharing stories and memories, and letting the person know how important they are to you.

• ***Saying good-bye.*** The dying process provides people with the opportunity to say good-bye to a person they love. Good-byes are challenging. They are also important. They're a chance to let people know what they have meant to each other and

> to acknowledge the role they've played in one another's lives.
>
> Good-byes are also opportunities to say other important things, like "Please forgive me" or "I forgive you," "Thank you" and, of course, "I love you." They can be an opportunity to address painful aspects of relationships. When a loved one is dying, asking for and offering forgiveness can be a powerful part of healing and moving forward. While there's no guarantee that you'll receive the response or acknowledgement that you expect or think you need, many people find some solace in knowing that they tried to address a painful part of their relationship.

I once worked with a young woman whose father was dying. The two had a very tumultuous relationship. One night, the week before her father died, she whispered in his ear, "I forgive you. We are good." Her father never responded. After he died, though, the daughter felt a great sense of peace, and she was happy that she had uttered those words at least once before he died. What mattered to her was that she truly forgave him. Saying "I forgive you" allowed her to let go of some of her long-held anger. That moment was integral to her grieving process and her eventual healing.

Good-byes also provide opportunities for expressions of gratitude. Thanking a person who is dying for being a part of your life contributes to their sense of dignity. People need to know that they made a difference in the lives of the people they touched and that their presence in the world mattered. When I said good-bye to Derrick, I thanked him for being a good friend, for being a significant and beloved adult in my children's lives, and for always being there when we needed him. I told him we would speak of him often, with love, and remember him always. I also told him that we'd be OK when he died and that we'd take care of one another—but that we would miss him awfully. Derrick's cancer often resulted in some difficult and undignified moments. I wanted him to know from my good-bye that he maintained his integrity and dignity as an important loved one in our lives.

We tend to think that good-byes need to be momentous occasions. In reality, if you are actively engaged in holding space for someone who is dying, you may say good-bye several times as your loved one moves through the dying process. Still, try not to wait until the last minute to say the things that you want to say. When death is near, make an effort to end each conversation as though it might be your last with that person—you want to know that you'll feel OK if it turns out to be the last time that you speak. A good-bye doesn't have to be mushy. You don't have to plan it out in advance. It can simply be the way in which you let the person know that they matter to you now and always will.

Remember that the person you are saying good-bye to will likely be saying good-bye to many, many people. This is difficult and emotional work. Added to the already momentous task of dying, it means that your loved one may not have the energy to match your heartfelt or emotional good-bye with the same level of emotion. Don't fret about this. It has nothing to do with the love you have shared.

You can say good-bye to a person who is no longer conscious. This may feel like a one-sided conversation. Many people who work in palliative care, however, believe that hearing is the last sense to go. While a loved one may be unresponsive, we believe that they are still able to hear. Sometimes, at this point, people wait for permission to die. A family member might, for example, say something like "It's OK to go now, Mom," or "We love you and we'll miss you, but we know you're tired. It's OK to leave us now." Sometimes the person who is dying needs to hear that those they love will be all right without them.

Leaving a Legacy

Holding space for someone you love as they die is not easy work. Caregivers often talk about how helpless they feel and how they "just want to do something." This is when it can be useful to think about creating a legacy.

Sometimes people get scared off by the idea of a "legacy." It sounds big and exorbitant. We may think of legacies as significant financial contributions to an institution like a hospital or university, or to a local arts organization.

While these are all wonderful ways to create legacies, they do not have to involve a large financial commitment—or any financial commitment at all, for that matter. A legacy is simply something we leave behind that shows that we lived and that we were loved. It is an intentional act designed to secure connection and memories. Legacy projects may help loved ones reminisce and share memories. They may also result in a tangible product that can be enjoyed after the person has died, but that is not necessary. Or it may be an activity that celebrates the dying person's life. However it's structured, the focus of legacy work is on life and living. It encourages people to connect and facilitates the sharing of important moments.

Opportunities for legacy projects are unlimited and as unique as the individuals in whose honour they are created. It might involve writing letters to loved ones, making a video recording, putting together a photo album or scrapbooks of memories. My uncle interviewed his father once a month after he was diagnosed with a terminal illness, recording the stories about his life in the "old country" and how he had immigrated to Canada. This project provided three generations with a deeper understanding of where their family had come from.

I had the privilege of supporting a pregnant woman while her own mother was dying in hospice. What a juxtaposition, to watch a baby grow inside this woman while the woman's mother slowly died. One of the daughter's biggest sorrows was knowing that her mom would never meet her new grandchild. The woman who was dying had a strong love of cooking and had shared a number of closely held family recipes with her daughter after her terminal diagnosis. As a legacy project, the daughter created a recipe box for her unborn child that contained all her mother's famous recipes. She sat bedside as her mother slept and painstakingly wrote out the recipes by hand. She recorded her memories of the occasions at which these dishes had been made and served, and words of advice to ensure their success. The recipe box became an essential connection between the new grandchild and the grandmother she would never meet.

Being There at the End

The moment of dying—that specific time when a dying person makes the transition from life to death—carries a great deal of weight in our culture. Many people think it is vitally important to be present for that moment. They worry that they will miss it and that their loved one will have died alone. If this happens, they can become devastated and feel as though they've let down the person they loved in their final moments.

It is important to remember that dying, like caregiving, is a process. People can hover between life and death for hours, and often days, and it is easy to miss the final moment. If you are not in the room with a loved one at the precise moment when he or she dies, that's not a sign that you were not a good caregiver. Nor does it negate your love for the person, or your grief at their death. It simply means that you missed one of many moments along the continuum from life to death. If you're worried that you will miss the final moments of a loved one's death, it can help to make sure that you have already said your good-byes and anything else important to you. If you have done so, you can take comfort in knowing that nothing was left unsaid. If you find yourself in this situation, remember to be gentle with yourself. It can also help to know that many people prefer to die alone.

A Solitary Death

Sometimes people will want to die alone. They may not want their loved ones to witness a moment that they regard as an unnecessary burden or heartache. Many people want to be remembered as being strong and active—they don't want many people to see them in their final days. When I worked in a hospice unit, I often saw parents, in particular, seemingly "choose" to die in the few moments that their children had left the room. It seemed as though they wanted to protect their children, regardless of their age, from the difficult things in life.

I remember one daughter who kept vigil at her mother's bedside 24 hours a day for almost a week. The daughter understood that her mother could die any moment, and she wanted to be there. One evening, the daughter left for fewer than 10 minutes, to go to the washroom and grab a glass of water. When she returned, her mother had died. We, the staff, were surprised. There were no signs that death was that imminent. We worried that the daughter would be distraught about having missed the death, but the daughter surprised us. She just sighed and said, "Always protecting me, eh, Mom?"

Signs of Death

It is almost impossible to predict when death will happen. Several physical clues, however, let us know that the time is near. These include

- Breathing changes: Sometimes a person will pant a few times as the heart and lungs stop working. People may take several long breaths with long intervals between them as the body shuts down. Sometimes people nearby find this hard to watch, as it may appear the person is struggling. It can help to know that this is the way the lungs expel air as they stop functioning.
- Body temperature will change, leaving the skin cool, warm, moist or pale.
- They may no longer be taking in any food or fluid.

- There may be different sleep-wake patterns.
- There will be fewer and smaller bowel movements and less urination.
- The person may be confused or seem to be in a daze.
- They may report seeing or being visited by people who have died.
- There may be movements or talking from the person who is dying that we do not understand.

Signs of death can also be psychological. It's not unusual, for example, for dying people to talk about wanting to "go home." In most cases, they want to return to their bricks-and-mortar home. Where possible, facilitate this visit. If a visit home isn't possible, get creative: bring pieces of home to the person who is dying. This may take the form of a favourite blanket or pillow, photographs, even a visit from the family pet.

But sometimes, people who are dying will express a desire to "go home" even when they are already at home. This might mean they want to return to a period in their life when they felt "at home" in their body and when life felt more normal and grounded. It could also mean that they are done living. They're ready to leave their physical body and move on to whatever follows. This interpretation views "home" in a spiritual sense and can be taken as an understanding that death is coming.

How can you respond to this spiritual request to "go home"? A good approach is to acknowledge and accept the request, and to offer reassurance that all will be well and they can let go of this life peacefully. It's not easy to do, but giving someone permission to "let go" and die is a meaningful act. It is not unusual for people to report that their loved one died in a peaceful way after they were told it was OK to let go.

People who are dying often report seeing someone who has already died. Sometimes the dying person will say they see a loved one or group of loved ones who have died standing at the window, near their bed or peering in the doorway. Sometimes, those people have a message of reassurance: they want the dying person to know that the next stop on their journey is ready, that it's a good place, or not to be scared.

These kinds of "supernatural" experiences don't often distress the person who is dying, but they can be very distressing for those who care for them. Sometimes caregivers worry that their loved one has taken too much pain medication or is hallucinating. Your healthcare team can help to assess this. Often, caregivers will tell the dying person that he or she is mistaken and only imagining things. It's best, however, not to argue, especially if seeing these people seems to comfort the dying person. Continue the positive tone by encouraging the person to feel comforted in the thought that loved ones are waiting to see and help them along the transition to death.

The Moment of Death, and What Follows

Sometimes the dying process can feel as though it takes a very long time. At other times, it can feel like it all happened so fast. But when death comes, most of us will know what is happening.

If you are sitting close to someone as they die, you will note that they are no longer breathing. You will see changes in the skin tone and temperature as blood stops circulating. The facial expression may seem to relax. Perhaps the most powerful sensation when a loved one moves from living to dead is the strong sense that the person they knew and loved is no longer there. Just the shell of the body has been left behind.

Many of us have expectations of the moment of death. We hope that it will be a spiritual experience. And some people do have that. For others, it is a time of mixed emotions. Some people may feel an instant rush of grief. Others feel numb and disconnected, or relieved. Sometimes it's a mixture of things. Witnessing someone else's death can cause us to consider our own mortality: we may find ourselves asking big questions about what life means to us as we work to figure out how the death of our loved one will affect our daily lives. The experience may alter how we now understand the world around us. But there is no right way to feel at this time. Everyone grieves differently.

After a person dies, whether the death takes place at home or in a hospital, long-term care facility or hospice, there's no rush to do anything. Take a moment, think about what has just happened, say another good-bye. Spend some time with the body if that feels right: many people report finding this important and often peaceful. Often, others will want to come and have a chance to say another good-bye. If possible, open a window to clear the air. Some people also believe that this allows the spirit to leave, and they find comfort in this thought.

Caring for Those Who Care

Dying is difficult. Being a caregiver for someone at the end of life can likewise be physically, emotionally and spiritually exhausting. If you're a caregiver, a person intimately involved, either formally or informally, with caring for a person who is dying, it's important to acknowledge the challenges of your role and to take care of yourself. This is easier said than done. Most people have other obligations—children, aging parents, work and managing a home—that require attention and energy. It's easy to forget about your own needs while you're pouring all your energy into caretaking and meeting other obligations. But if you don't take care of yourself, you risk your own health and, in turn, compromise your ability to be there for the person who is dying. Simply put, it is very difficult to care for someone else when you aren't taking care of yourself. As writer, artist and gerontologist Eleanor Brownn writes, "Self-care is not selfish. You cannot serve from an empty vessel."

Looking after yourself can take many forms. Here are some suggestions:

> ***Take breaks.*** Eat a nutritious meal, have a nap, take a bath or go for a walk. If it's important to you that someone is always with the dying person, organize shifts with other family members and friends so you know who will be sitting vigil. Hospice volunteers can also help here—ask your health-care team for information about hospice services. If your loved one is at home and you need to keep track of them, use a baby monitor or other technology so you can keep in contact while you are in another room.

> ***Accept help from others.*** Sometimes it's hard to accept help from others. Caregivers may feel needy or inadequate if they ask for help from other people who are close to the dying person. Keep in mind that most people truly want to help. They, too, feel helpless as they face the death of someone they care about, and are often happy and relieved to be of service, even in some small way. Accept offers of help and give specific suggestions when people ask what they can do. They can shop for groceries, mow the lawn, walk

the dog, return library books, give children lifts to lessons and activities, sit with the person who is dying while you take a break, or just come for a visit.

Pay attention to your sleep and nutrition. As a caregiver, you're used to monitoring your loved one's sleeping and eating patterns. Don't forget about your own. Eat regularly and well (and no, take-out coffee and doughnuts don't count as "eating well") and get enough sleep. Otherwise, your own health will suffer. You can request a cot if you are spending nights in the hospital, and consider bringing your own pillows and blankets so you might sleep better. Let others who want to help bring you food or spell you off so you can have a good night's sleep.

Experiencing the death of someone you love is never easy. As a caretaker, though, some the pain of loss may be eased in the knowledge that you were needed and that you stepped up and did what you could to care for your loved one.

CHAPTER EIGHT

Posting, Tweeting & Texting: Dying and Death in a Digital World

"Social media is not a media. The key is to listen, engage, and build relationships."
—David Alston, Digital Society Advocate

Kate Granger was diagnosed with cancer in July of 2011. Over the course of her illness and, eventually, her death at the age of 34, Granger—an English geriatrician—took to social media to champion better and more compassionate care from hospital staff and increased visibility and transparency around the dying process. Her #hellomynameis Twitter campaign encouraged medical personnel to perform a simple yet radically human act—to introduce themselves, by name, to the people they cared for. As she explained, "I firmly believe it is not just about common courtesy, but it runs much deeper. Introductions are about making a human connection between one human being who is suffering and vulnerable, and another human being who wishes to help. They begin therapeutic relationships and can instantly build trust in difficult circumstances." The campaign was endorsed by more than 400,000 doctors, nurses, therapists, receptionists and other hospital and health-care workers across the United Kingdom and beyond. Granger's hashtag has made over 1 billion impressions since its inception, with an average of six tweets an hour. As her illness progressed and it became clear that she wouldn't recover, Granger decided to live-tweet her dying process, using the hashtag #deathbedlive as part of her efforts to normalize discussions about dying and death. At the time of her death, on July 23, 2016, she had just shy of 50,000 Twitter followers. That number has continued to grow.

Most of Granger's online followers never met her offline. Still, thousands of them were saddened by the news of her death and took to Twitter to share their thoughts, memories and gratitude for her contributions. She helped them understand better the concept of "living until you die," and about using social media as a tool not only for advocacy and change but as a way to demystify and understand the dying process and our feelings around it.

Not everyone facing a terminal illness can live out loud online the way @GrangerKate did. But people have always used the tools available to them to express sorrow and grief, to tell stories of those who have died and to make sure our loved ones are not forgotten. In the past, people have faced death and dying through drawings on caves or embalming mummies, through art or obituaries in the newspaper, through photographs, donations and charity runs. Today, the digital world presents us with considerable new and innovative ways to share and engage others in our experiences of dying, death and grief. North Americans have turned to platforms like Twitter, Facebook and Instagram to talk about dying and death, posting their updates alongside food photos, trending memes and vacation shots.

Social media now often takes a leading role in spreading news about diagnoses and deaths. It shapes the way we offer support and provide education for people who are dying and those who love them. It even shapes how we are remembered after we die. Social media is changing—and expanding—the way we think, talk and engage with each other about the end of life.

That may be a good thing. Increased online exposure to death and dying gives us opportunities to learn about death from the virtual safety of our computers and digital devices. It brings conversations about illness and death out of the closet and into the light, acclimatizing us to the idea that death is part of life. Social media can make communication around death and dying more immediate, continuous and succinct. But it can also raise doubts or uncomfortable feelings for some people. And they may find themselves not emotionally prepared to deal with the posts and tweets that come their way.

However much social media does good work in normalizing our conversations around death, it does raise questions of etiquette and propriety. Are there some things that just should not be shared via email or text? Are there messages that require only in-person communication? There is no right answer to these questions. It depends on the individuals involved. Some people could not bear to know that such personal news about them was out in cyberspace. Others would find it an efficient and effective method of communication. Still others would take advantage of more private and dedicated sites, which I will talk about next.

Sharing about Illness

Not too long ago, if a person became seriously ill or was diagnosed with a terminal illness, they often faced social isolation and loneliness alongside their deteriorating health. In just a few generations, we had lost the ability to talk easily about these topics as medical advances insulated us against the day-to-day reality of frequent and untimely death. And people certainly didn't have a platform at their fingertips that allowed them to provide status updates and photographs of their doctor's appointments, bedside visitors or recovery room shots to a virtually unlimited audience, should they choose to do so. Technology lets people who are ill create or join online communities that serve as safe spaces to share the challenges of their illnesses and their day-to-day experiences. Our comfort zone for sharing the personal details of our lives has broadened to the point where even illness, death and grief are fair game. Some have even tweeted updates of their loved ones' dying process. But where are the privacy lines that we should not cross? Do they even still exist?

When I found out I had cancer, I wanted to rally family and friends for support and love. I wanted to keep them updated, but I also needed to save my energy. Email could have been an acceptable option, but my husband and I decided to use a website called CaringBridge.org—what I fondly referred to as "Facebookfor sick people." CaringBridge.org is a private, ad-free site that encourages ill people to invite trusted family and friends to a dedicated online space. On this site, they update friends and family on their illness and develop a supportive community *that they can control.* The website gave me an opportunity to tell my story one time, instead of individually to every single friend or family member who cared about me. Given that I was physically and emotionally exhausted, I appreciated not having to repeat the same, often emotionally charged, information over and over. The platform also allowed me to control the information about my illness: I shared only what I wanted, with whom I wanted, and I never worried that I'd mistakenly left someone off the email list. I knew that those who joined my Caring Bridge online community would go to my page when they chose. I didn't worry about bombarding them with too much information, because they too could control how often they looked at my site.

And I loved the support I received. In the same way that people use Facebook, my chosen online community would write on my "wall" and send private messages. Sometimes old friends who had lost touch with one another actually reconnected through the site. My husband and I could look at it any time we felt scared, lonely or needed a pick-me-up. And when I, thankfully, no longer had a use for the site, when I returned home and was well on the way to recovery, I closed and deleted my account. But before I did that, I printed off all the messages of support, the pictures, the jokes and the updates my husband and I posted as a record of that challenging time in my life. I bound them together as a keepsake of the time I threw my net wide on an online platform and asked for and received support from a fabulous community. Making a keepsake of the items friends and family have posted on a closed site like this can also provide support and fond mementos after a loved one has died. It can act much like the online condolence books that funeral homes are now using.

Grief

Picture it: you're scrolling through your Facebook feed, as one does, past back-to-school or Halloween pictures, or shots of someone's most recent gourmet meal. And then you read an update—your friend's mother has died. Or maybe an acquaintance's father has been taken ill. Or a friend's toddler has been diagnosed with a devastating illness. What do you do? How do you respond? Do you feel empathy, compassion? Or do you feel like a voyeur, uncomfortably indulging in somebody else's personal life? Can you pretend that you didn't see the post? Can you "like" a post that talks about a death in the family? Is it OK to share the post to make sure that your mutual Facebook friends know, too? Is it acceptable to express support and condolences as a comment after someone's post? If you do, should you still send a sympathy card?

The etiquette on these types of online interactions is evolving almost as quickly as the web itself. The web can be a way to reach out or to distance ourselves, to offer meaningful support or what may feel like shallow overtures. It can ease our sense of isolation or magnify it. Like any other tool, we can use social media and other technology in ways that are productive and supportive in the face of death and illness, or we can use them in ways that aren't helpful.

I recently learned of the death of a friend's father through a Facebook posting. I had gone to her Facebook page looking for a vacation update and instead came across a post from someone I didn't know. The post was a bit vague, but I was pretty sure that something serious had happened to my friend's father. I decided not to post on my friend's page, because she's not on Facebook all that much. Instead, I texted her, *Heard about your dad. I'm here. How can I help? xo.* The response came back almost immediately. *Of course you'd figure it out. Didn't have a chance to call—can't talk about it yet and am getting on a plane. Thanks for letting me know you know.* Technology allowed me to reach out and offer support in a way that traditional methods would not have. Most likely my friend would not have answered a phone call as she was rushing to catch a plane. Even if she had time to answer, knowing her, she wouldn't have wanted to risk crying in public, which may well have happened on the phone. Texting was safe. Short and to the point from both of us. We initiated a connection that acknowledged the event, and we knew we could talk more intimately in the future. And, importantly, we did.

Deathiquette and Netiquette

We are still navigating the waters around dying, death, grief and loss online. How can we do so most appropriately? Often, it's a case of applying the same standards to social media as we do in "real-life" (no pun intended) situations. Here's what I would suggest:

> ***Acknowledge the loss.*** It's generally considered acceptable to comment on a post about death or illness. If a person risks declaring online that someone important to them has died, acknowledge it. Ideally, you would write a short post

acknowledging the loss and offering your condolences. For example, you could say: "Sue was such a dynamic person. We will really miss her in our book club. Please accept my condolences and know I'm thinking of you."

It's OK to not know what to say. Many of us become tongue-tied when we learn about someone's death. Sometimes our words feel inadequate amid the immensity of the situation. It is perfectly acceptable to admit that words fail you. For example, you could write, "I heard about your dad. I'm so sorry. I really don't know what else to say, but I wanted you to know I'm thinking of you and sending love." This kind of response communicates that you still want to show up and acknowledge that something important has happened and that you care. Admitting that you don't know what to say is always preferable to relying on pithy statements or sometimes hurtful platitudes such as "At least he's in peace now" or "Your child was so perfect, God wanted her to sit beside him."

If you're still at a loss for words, you can choose from one of several emoticons Facebook has recently provided, including a thumbs-up, a heart, a laughing face, a face that appears shocked, one with a tear and a face that appears angry. For the many of us who (probably rightly) felt hesitant to "like" a post about death, this expanded menu of options is particularly helpful when someone writes that a loved one has died. These emoticons and their meaning are open to interpretation. Most people will probably choose the face with the tear to communicate sadness upon learning the news. Some people may choose the heart to express their love for the person who died and/or the person who shared the news.

Follow up. Depending on your relationship with either the person who has died or the person who wrote the post, you may consider following up with a direct message, sharing a memory or making a specific offer of support, such as a visit, going to the funeral or dropping off a meal. It is important that our online posts, be they public or private, follow the same sort of standards we might have in person. For example, if upon hearing of the death of a friend's parent you would hug them when you saw them in person, you can also make this offer of support online. Very simply, this could be a post like: "Heard about your mom. Sending a big hug. Hope to see you in person soon."

Make sure it's not about you. Post an expression of support to the person who made the original post, not a statement about you. It is not helpful for the person sharing the news to know how shocked you are and that you don't think you can go to work because you are too devastated. Avoid the temptation to suggest that you know what the other person is going through. Grief is an individual experience. While you may have also experienced the death of a loved one, the person you are attempting to support has his or her own, individual experience. Keep your experiences to yourself initially—at least until you are asked to share.

If it's not your news, don't share it. If someone has died, take a moment to see how those most closely involved with that person share the news. Allow them to choose whether they would like to use social media to share this information or not. And then, respect that decision. If a person has announced a death, it's a good idea to ask their permission before sharing the news publicly on your own page.

Use the "D" words! Straight talk is important here. Don't hide behind euphemisms or watered-down phrases—like *expired, passed on* or *lost*—that attempt to ignore the reality of the experience of death. The milk in my fridge expires; people die—it is very different. Don't be afraid to use the D words—*dead, died* or *death.* This is particularly important if you are communicating in a post or tweet whose platform requires a brevity that may almost seem curt or disrespectful. You will not cause any more pain to a grieving person by using straightforward language that acknowledges their reality. It is a sign of respect.

Use social networking to enhance support, not replace it. For some, dealing with death and grief via social media may be more comfortable than real-life interactions. Facebook, Twitter and other online platforms allow them to share information and receive support and acknowledgement in a more controlled environment. But that's not the case for all of us. Sometimes grieving people don't feel as though they've received the support and recognition they expected from their online community. Perhaps they didn't receive as many responses as they expected. Perhaps the quality of those responses didn't feel as supportive and caring as they might have in face-to-face interactions.

Especially with close friends and family members, don't let social networking platforms replace the face-to-face support and conversation we still need while we're grieving. Consider what you would expect and want from certain people in the event that you experienced the death of a loved one. Give that back to them.

Funerals and Memorials

Part of the work of grief is to maintain a continuing bond with the person who has died. Today's technology provides us with many different options to do so in the virtual world.

For example, it has become almost expected for funeral homes to offer live streaming of the funeral service for those who are unable to attend in person. Video tributes, online guest books and web-based memorial sites have added additional layers of opportunity for people to share condolences. These online spaces let people post stories, photos, videos and narratives at any time of day or night, at minimal cost, as often as they want. They allow us to make donations with the click of a mouse. They are a new kind of hieroglyphic, a form of writing on the wall, to tell the tale of those we have loved who have died.

If technology has changed the way we gather to remember our dead and support our loved ones, it also mirrors grief rituals we've performed and participated in through time and across cultures. In Mexico, for example, baked sweets and favoured possessions of the dead are left on altars to honour the departed. This ritual reminds me of how Facebook members share cherished memories, stories and favourite photos on the timelines of friends who have died. Let's use our newfound technology to expand the range of rituals that help us continue a connection with the person who has died and allow us to grieve. But remember, for many, these technologies do not replace personal connection and support.

Your Digital Legacy

A friend of mine died unexpectedly last year. In the week after the incident that ultimately ended his life, his profile page served as an outlet for friends, colleagues and acquaintances to get updates on his condition and express their support and love for him. After his death, the page turned into a place to inform people about his death, share memories and stories, offer condolences and make plans for his funeral.

Today, when I visited my friend's Facebook page, I saw acknowledgements of his recent birthday, recognitions of the anniversary of his death and gestures of kindness toward his wife. One friend even posted a note about a recent success that he knew my friend would have loved to hear about. The traffic on my friend's page is decreasing. I don't visit it very often these days, but I do like to stop by occasionally to look at his picture, read some posts and think about and miss him in my everyday life. I don't know why his wife hasn't removed her husband's page, but I'm grateful that it's still accessible.

There are many reasons to keep Facebook, Twitter, Instagram or other social media accounts open or active even after their owner has died. These accounts can act as memorials or testaments. They can act as a virtual scrapbook of memories, important life events and interactions with people who cared about the person. These virtual memorials are certainly more convenient than visiting a cemetery for many of us. There is no need to get into a car and drive anywhere. Most of us have easy access to a computer, where a friend's smiling profile picture is only a click away.

Not everyone thinks it's a good idea to keep online profiles active after their owners have died. Profiles can show up under the "people you know" feature; friends of the deceased may receive reminders of upcoming birthdays. For some, these reminders may hurt or even be spooky—as if they are receiving a message from the dead. People who haven't heard about the death may attempt to get in touch or offer birthday greetings. These kinds of situations can at best be socially awkward. At worst, they cause pain.

Most North Americans haven't thought about what happens to their social media accounts when they die or become too ill to manage them. Few of us have plans in place for our loved ones to delete, manage or memorialize our accounts. For all the above reasons, though, we need to think about our own and our loved ones' digital legacies. What do you want to happen to your online profile when you die? What will your online legacy be? In the same way that we think about how we want our property and possessions to be handled after we die, we need to consider our digital footprints as well.

In this evolving arena, we can do a few things to make this a bit easier for those charged with closing up our estates after we die. First, leave some direction for the executor. Make a list of your social media accounts and their passwords. Specify how you would like each account to be handled after you die. Maybe you would like a loved one or trusted friend or colleague to send one last tweet on your behalf. Perhaps you want to change your LinkedIn account to "permanently retired." Facebook now offers its users the option of having an account "memorialized" or permanently deleted after a death, and users can appoint someone to manage their account through its Legacy Contact feature.

Our online presence is always changing as different forums and platforms come onto the scene or become obsolete. (Myspace, anyone?) Keep your list up to date and make sure your executor knows where it is.

Think about your digital farewell. Just as it has become more popular and accepted for people to help plan their own funerals or celebrations of life, or to write their own obituaries, it is becoming and will become more common for people to send out messages of farewell or notices of death via social media. Slowly, people are using these platforms as a chance to acknowledge their impending death and to say good-bye.

As you begin to consider your digital legacy, you may find the following questions useful as conversation-starters with your loved ones:

- How do you feel about loved ones posting information about you on social media in the days leading up to and following your death? Would you want them to chronicle your dying process? Would it be OK to post pictures of you in the hospital, or of your family?
- Would you want information about your funeral or memorial service to be posted online? What about your obituary?
- Would you like your Facebook and other social media accounts to continue after your death, would you like them to be converted to memorial sites if that's an option or would you like them removed? Who has access to these accounts?

As we share more information on digital platforms, let's strive to communicate about dying and death in the ways that serve us best. Let us continue to recognize that death and dying are an integral part of life and living, and that they have a place on our Facebook walls or Twitter feeds along with birth announcements and vacation pictures. Let us reach out to one another in a supportive way, knowing that one day we may be posting or tweeting about the death of our own loved one and looking for acknowledgement and caring responses. Let us, like Kate Granger, continue to make the online world a safe and open place to learn about and support one another through illness, dying, death and grief.

CHAPTER NINE

Dying on (Some of) Our Own Terms

"Death has been moved out of nature into human responsibility."
—Daniel Callahan, biomedical ethicist and author

"Just get me a pine box"; "I want a pine box." Those two phrases are what I remember of a man, John, dying of a terminal illness on the hospice unit where I worked. I am not exaggerating when I say that was all John said for the two weeks it took him to die. He was ready for his life to be over and death was not coming quickly enough. It was challenging for everyone involved in John's care. As palliative-care providers, we wanted to support him and make him comfortable to the best of our abilities, without either hastening or prolonging his life. John's family was tired and sad, and appeared devastated that he only wanted his life to end. When he actually did die, we all shared feelings of guilt and inadequacy, wishing we could have done something different so that John's last few weeks were not so hard, and so that the memories of those who loved him would not be so permanently tainted by the continual plea for a pine box.

The landscape that Canadians now die in has changed in the years following John's death. It is almost impossible to discuss dying and death in Canada now without including MAID. MAID stands for "medical assistance in dying" and is the official term for medically hastened death. On February 6, 2015, the Supreme Court of Canada sent down a decision regarding *Carter v. Canada* legalizing physician-assisted death. This was a landmark decision that changed the prohibition of doctors helping terminally ill patients end their own lives. The court concluded that such a prohibition was against the Canadian Charter of Rights and Freedoms.

There were a number of people leading this challenge, including Kay Carter, a woman suffering from degenerative spinal stenosis, and Gloria Taylor, living with amyotrophic lateral sclerosis (ALS). The Supreme Court decision was unanimous and struck down the provision in the Criminal Code of Canada that made a physician's assistance in a terminally ill person's suicide a criminal act. This decision has given Canadian adults who are mentally competent, suffering intolerably and facing a reasonably imminent death the right to a medically hastened ending. The court was responding to Canadians' changing attitudes to the issue, and its decision recognized that a majority of Canadians have expressed a strong desire for choice and autonomy over the way they die. This decision will have an impact on how we talk about dying and death in this country, and how we talk to our families and our health-care providers as we think about the way we wish to be treated at the end of our lives.

Unpacking the Terms

Medical assistance in dying (MAID) in Canada is also known as physician-assisted suicide or medically hastened death. It's an option to citizens who are considered capable of making an informed decision, have a diagnosis of a life-limiting illness, are suffering unbearably from that illness as it progresses and are seen to have a "reasonably foreseeable" death. MAID involves a physician or nurse practitioner—no other health practitioners in Canada are permitted to do this—directly administering or prescribing a specific formula of death-causing medication to an individual at their request. It is the role of the pharmacist to dispense the prescription. The federal legislation spells out two methods that may be followed. The physician or nurse practitioner can administer a medication through an intravenous or another method intended to hasten death directly. Or they prescribe or provide the medication cocktail to the individual to self-administer orally at a later time. Other health-care professionals, such as nurses or social workers, can provide information to a person on how medical assistance in dying is permitted in Canada. The federal legislation also permits individuals, such as a family member, to help a patient self-administer the necessary drugs, provided that the patient explicitly requests the individual's help. In Canada, specifically in Ontario, for example the drugs required to medically hasten death are covered by the government at no additional expense to the individual.

It is important to emphasize that MAID is only conducted at the specific request of an individual who is mentally competent to make the decision. Competency, or capability, is determined by ensuring the individual understands what they are requesting and the implications of their actions. Presently in Canada, the legislation requires that the terminally ill individual expressly consent to hastening their death immediately before MAID is provided. One cannot request MAID before death is "reasonably foreseeable," even if the illness might eventually make it difficult or impossible for the person to consent before an assisted death, for example when an individual is diagnosed with dementia. Family members or friends cannot act as substitute decision-makers and have no legal authority to consent to or authorize MAID on behalf of an individual.

This legislation has been controversial, as it means that Canadians living with dementia who may have expressed a desire to hasten their death do not qualify for this intervention if they are not found capable at the time MAID might be implemented. This may change in the future, as the current federal legislation requires the Canadian government to conduct a mandatory review after two years to ascertain if allowing advance medical directives for MAID will be feasible and appropriate in the future.

It is the request made by a capable and informed individual that differentiates MAID from euthanasia. In the act of euthanasia, a person knowingly and intentionally (usually without consent from the individual) ends the life of a person who has an incurable illness. There is an important distinction between euthanasia and murder. With euthanasia, the person who ends another's life acts with empathy and compassion, and without personal gain, and the person whose life has been ended has an illness without a cure.

The term medical assistance in dying is somewhat controversial within the palliative-care community. This is because many healthcare professionals working in palliative and end-of-life care would argue that the care they provide *is* medical assistance in dying, just not as narrowly defined as in the new legislation. What palliative-care providers offer does not hasten or prolong death; it strives to relieve pain and suffering and supports the natural process of dying as a normative life event. The medical assistance comes from the palliative-care team in the form of medical assessment, medication for symptom relief, knowledge and treatment; pain and symptom management; and psychosocial and spiritual care. What MAID offers actively hastens death by pharmaceutical means. The important difference is that palliative and end-of-life care promote naturally occurring death and the assistance provided neither intentionally hastens death nor prolongs life.

Palliative-care providers, in tandem with the people they are caring for, may make decisions to withhold or withdraw life-sustaining interventions that could include such treatment as dialysis, artificial ventilation and nutrition and feeding. Such decisions are generally made because the treatment may no longer be worthwhile, or because the individual receiving the treatment no longer wishes it. While these decisions eventually result in death, this is not the same as MAID. Which is why from now on in this book, I will mostly refer to MAID as medically hastened death.

Why Someone Might Request a Medically Hastened Death

As I have said often through this book, dying is hard work. It tends not to be a smooth, linear process that we can anticipate. It often entails suffering, vulnerability, pain and loneliness. It is understandable, then, that dying is not a life event most of us embark upon willingly.

Some of the specific reasons that someone might request medically hastened death are not that different from why many of us are fearful of dying and death. Some request it because they want to maintain a sense of control and autonomy. Others may find the suffering they are experiencing is too great to bear and want to end their suffering. Still others view their dying as a burden on their families and do not want it to continue. Pain and poor symptom-management used to be a reason that people who were dying would request to end their lives. But today, with the advancements in medication, knowledge of pain and symptom-management, and with access to palliative and end-of-life care, this need no longer to be a reason to seek medically hastened death.

Sometimes people assume that the person who is dying is clinically depressed if they request MAID. However, research has shown that the psychosocial distress involved with dying—including feeling like a burden, lacking social support, spiritual distress and a deteriorating quality of life—tends to be the decisive factor.

From a distance, dying appears to be about only loss and suffering. However, many people who have helped care for a dying person whose pain and symptoms are controlled have found that this can be an intense and rewarding experience for those involved. It can be a time that allows for meaningful communication and valuable time spent together. Medically hastened death and euthanasia both offer an immediate end to suffering, and that makes them seem attractive options to some when life is coming to an end.

It is important to continue to discuss, examine and improve how we care for people at the end of their lives. The way we treat our most vulnerable members of society says a lot about what we value. Having options at the end of life that include access to palliative and end-of-life care for all Canadians will help ensure that people die a death that is congruent with their personal values.

These end-of-life decisions are not binary. A medically hastened death does not always mean that a person has a dignified death. A good or appropriate death can also be achieved when pain and other symptoms are well-managed and controlled, when psychosocial support and spiritual care are provided, and when the dying process is recognized as a valued part of life and living. It will be a paradigm shift in thinking about death should Canadians come to a place where they consider their dying to be a part of their life legacy rather than just the end of it.

Discussing the Option of Hastening Death with Your Health-Care Provider

It is not uncommon for people with advanced illness to ask questions about hastening death or to express their readiness to die. This has been happening more frequently in the months since the MAID legislation was passed. A person's desires may change as the months or years of their illness pass, or as their experience of living in the shadow of their death alters. Still, to date only about 10 percent of people with a life-limiting illness consider hastening their death, and an even lower percentage actually pursues it with a health-care provider or physician. For example, in the state of Oregon, where physician-assisted suicide has been legalized since 1997 and is readily available, only .002 percent of the total deaths in 2012 occurred through medically hastened death.

It is never too early to have discussions with your physician and health-care providers. As MAID is new in Canada and the processes required to access the service are still being established and under trial in most communities, it is important to discuss your end-of-life wishes with your doctor as early as possible. There will be different procedures in each province. Your health-care providers should be aware of the process that is appropriate for you.

Presently in Canada, the option for conscientious objection is still available for health-care providers. This means that yours are not required to offer you medically hastened death as an option, nor to prescribe the required medications or be present for the hastened death. Should your physician be opposed to medically hastened death, they should be prepared to refer you to someone who isn't. There is an expectation in the province of Ontario, for example, that the referral will be made in a timely manner and in good faith to a non-objecting, available and accessible physician to complete the intervention.

Your family and friends may be initially upset by your desire for a hastened death and unprepared to have the discussion with you. If your health-care provider has an understanding of your thoughts and preferences in this area, they can support you in planning for the death that is most appropriate for your values and condition, and they can act as an advocate on your behalf. A suggestion for initiating this conversation might look like something like this: "If I were terminally ill and wanted to end my life by MAID, would you be willing to support me in this?" Should your physician respond "no," the follow-up would be to request a referral to a physician who would be willing, an obligation your physician will fulfill to the best of their abilities.

MAID is constantly in the news, so physicians should not be surprised if the topic comes up with their patients during appointments. The legislation has changed the options for Canadians at the end of their lives, and physicians are at the forefront of this change. Perhaps the best time for this conversation is during your routine visits with your family physician, when you discuss changes in health, update advance care plans and talk about preferred treatment.

As with most things pertaining to care at the end of life, the discussion involving medically hastened death will be an evolving process, but it is important to lay the proper foundations as early as possible. You can begin the conversation by letting your physician know you have been paying attention to the news and changes in Canadian legislation and that you want to be prepared. In the same way that you can share your thoughts about your advance care plans, you can tell your physician what is important to you and that you would like to make sure he or she understands and is willing to act according to your wishes in this important issue.

A way to begin this conversation might be: "Quality of life is really important to me. We've talked about what gives me quality. If that is no longer present for me and the end of life looks like it will be nothing but suffering, I would like to have my death hastened with your support."

The responses that you receive may be varied. Ideally, you will hear with certainty that the physician or nurse practitioner will support your decision to hasten your death. Or you may hear that it is too soon to talk about that, or that a discussion of that nature would better occur when the issue is imminent, along with a promise to keep you comfortable and take care of you. If that happens, an appropriate reply might be: "I understand that I need to make the request to hasten my death immediately before MAID is provided, but I want you to know that I'm thinking that it will be a suitable request when the time comes. If that is an issue for you, please refer me to someone who will be able to support my request." Again, it is then your health-care provider's responsibility to make an appropriate and timely referral.

Discussing the Option of Hastening Death with Your Family

Each family is unique, and each will respond to a family member's desire to request medically hastened death differently. Currently in Canada, there is no formal notification process for families when an individual requests a medically hastened death or is provided with MAID. The way the legislation is structured means that it is the choice and responsibility of the individual who is requesting the intervention and, like other health-care interactions, the request is to be kept confidential. The information is only shared with the family should the individual making the request provide formal consent that it be. As the individual seeking MAID needs to be considered capable of making the decision at the time of the request, family members do not possess any right under the law to intervene.

Presently in Ontario there is no formal notification to inform a family if the death was hastened, but each hastened death is required to be reported to the Office of the Chief Coroner and will be investigated during the initial monitoring period of this new legislative practice.

Despite the legislation's protection of confidentiality, as with most things associated with dying and death, individuals are strongly encouraged to discuss their preferences and desire to pursue MAID with those closest to them and involve them in discussions with health-care providers. As well, the legislation allows for a family member or other designate to assist the person hastening their death in administering the required drugs, provided that the request is clearly made.

We do not yet have the research to inform us how Canadian families react to the medically hastened death of a loved one, or how it affects their grief. We know from other places where medically hastened death is also legalized, such as Oregon and Switzerland, that many family members understand and support their loved ones' requests to end their lives. Families have also reported meaningful involvement with the dying persons at the end of life, knowing their death came in a controlled and pain-free way. To date, there are minimal studies examining the bereavement experiences of family members who were not informed of their loved ones' decisions to pursue medically hastened death. It's an area that needs more research.

Many of us have a good idea what our family and close friends think about medically hastened death, and it is only to be expected that the opinions will be varied. Some will be supportive and believe that it is the individual's right to have the death they choose. Others may object strongly. Some may fear losing the person to death sooner than expected and cannot imagine life without that person. Other objections may be more ethical or religious in nature.

If a family member or close friend objects, acknowledge that you respect their feelings, that they do not have to approve, and that you are not asking for their permission. Ask the individual to respect your wishes by not interfering. Again, Canadian legislation is such that you do not need to inform anyone but your health-care provider and one additional uninvolved witness, someone who is not a beneficiary of your will, who can witness your consent, of your intent.

However, the reality is that this decision has the potential for complicating the grief process in ways that we do not yet understand. This is new territory that Canadians are navigating, so you will need to decide what is in the best interests of both you and your family. Organizations such as Dying with Dignity believe it is preferable that the person who is dying shares what they are planning with their family and friends, providing them with the option to accept or reject it and to work out personal and past differences. The opportunity to be informed and to understand what decisions were made can assist loved ones in coping with the grief and bereavement they will face after the death. And should they not find themselves able to support your decision, you will have made the effort to communicate your needs, fears and vision of what you would like your death to be. Letting them know your plans can support families and loved ones and help them rise to the occasion by learning to accept your decisions.

Concluding Thoughts

As unusual as it may sound, it is an exciting time to be working to improve how people die in Canada. If John was still alive today, I strongly suspect his last few weeks of life would be different. He might still ask for the "pine box," but his health-care team and his family would be able to have more productive conversations with him because we now have more options for how to end our lives. Perhaps John would have opted for a medically hastened death. Because of the legislation, he might have decided that it afforded him "peace of mind," as has been found in Oregon, and he would have been comfortable on our hospice unit and died naturally. Death would still have been the outcome, but most likely his family would have very different memories today.

Canadians have asked for choice at the end of life and now we have a new option, but it is important that we do not allow this new option to move us away from the work of constantly improving how we approach human suffering and care for people at the end of their lives. Most likely, few Canadians will ultimately choose MAID, but many of us will be thankful that we live in a society where it is an option. Therefore, it is critical that we also have access to high-quality palliative and end-of-life care regardless of geography or diagnosis. It is important that we continue to tell our legislators and government leaders that how we die matters. We want to have access to the best care possible in environments that allow us to have some autonomy and ownership of our dying process. People should be able to assume that when the time comes, they will have access to palliative-care expertise, including physical, psychosocial, existential and spiritual care that will support them and their families, regardless of the decisions they might make at the end of their lives. It is up to the healthy to make these expectations known, as those who are dying are often too ill to speak up, and the dead no longer complain. We, the living, must use our voices so that when our time comes, we will be dying in a society that understands that how we die matters. We need to see ourselves as active members of a society that values all stages of life and living, including death and dying. In the words of Dame Cicely Saunders (1918–2005), nurse, physician and writer, and founder of the hospice movement, "You matter because you are you, and you matter to the end of your life. We will do all we can not only to help you die peacefully, but also to live until you die."

CHAPTER TEN

Moving the Conversation Forward

"If you want others to be happy, practise compassion. If you want to be happy, practise compassion."
—The Dalai Lama

Death is not a medical event. It's a social process. Dying and death do not occur in a vacuum. How we learn about it is strongly influenced by our social and religious communities. Often these communities are a wealth of support and strength, but sometimes they need education and mobilization so that they can offer support to those who need it. It is time for Canadians to reclaim dying as a social process and remove it from the medical realm. A person who is dying spends only 5 to 10 percent of her time within the healthcare system, yet that is where we tend to focus most of our time and energy and resources. There are many initiatives worldwide striving to bring dying back into the community setting. We need to develop our communities as a place to live where dying matters.

Many of us want to improve the care of the dying and their families and to have more options for end-of-life care. Numerous researchers, advocacy groups, politicians, citizens and health-care organizations are working diligently to address the gaps in our system. In Canada, we have the Canadian Hospice Palliative Care Association, Hospice Palliative Care Ontario, end-of-life care networks, for example. Many would be shocked to learn there is still an overwhelming majority who die each year without receiving any palliative care. It has also been estimated that only 16 to 30 percent of Canadians have had any access to palliative care, and those who did generally had it only within the last days or weeks of life. This lack of access is recognized as the most serious public health-care issue in Canada, one that continues to worsen (CHPCA, 2012).

Public Health Palliative Care International insists on its website homepage that "death, dying, loss and care is everyone's responsibility," and the Canadian Medical Association is advocating for a national palliative-care strategy. Yet in current Canadian society, elderly persons often spend their last days in nursing homes, hospitals or extended-care facilities. As a result, many of their family members are not active, hands-on caregivers involved in their loved ones' dying, even if they are involved in care decisions. Many families no longer learn about dying and death through the provision of care for their loved ones at home, but this is changing. A growing number of Canadians are finding the value and meaning in being more involved in care of their loved ones at the end of life and are looking for more education and greater support to facilitate them doing this.

Nothing in life is more certain than death and the fact that we will encounter death throughout our lives. The longer we live, the more experiences we will have with death. Recognizing the universality of death as a shared life experience, and the health-care system's concentration on best-practice interventions throughout the continuum of life, it stands to reason that there is a need to inform citizens about healthy ways to die. So how do we do this?

What is a Compassionate Community?

"I live in a community where everybody recognizes that we all have a role to play in supporting each other in times of crisis and loss. People are ready, willing and content to have conversations about living and dying well and to support each other in emotional and practical ways."

—Ambitions for Palliative and End of Life Care: A National Framework for Local Action 2015–2020

Compassionate communities are grounded in a public-health approach to end-of-life care. The concept originated in the work of Professor Allan Kellehear, an Australian public-health academic. Aligning his thinking with a public-health approach, Dr. Kellehear reminded us that health is everyone's responsibility, and that this needs to also include death, dying and end-of-life care. His concept of a compassionate community is one that becomes a place of support and care for people and their families who are dying or living with loss. The goal is the opportunity for all of us to live well within our communities to the very end of our lives.

Dr. Kellehear, in his book *Compassionate Cities: Public Health and End-of-Life Care,* writes that some of the defining features of a compassionate community are:

- Local health policies that recognize compassion as an ethical imperative;
- Meeting the special needs of its aged, those living with life-threatening illnesses and those living with loss;
- A strong commitment to social and cultural differences;
- Grief and palliative care services in local government policy and planning;
- Access to a wider variety of supportive experiences, interactions and communication;
- Promoting and celebrating reconciliation with Indigenous peoples and memory of other important community losses;
- Providing easy access to grief and palliative-care services.

You can find examples of compassionate community initiatives in the resource list at the back of this book.

So what, then, should or could the landscape of dying and death for Canadians look like in the future? There is a shift happening now as many people are beginning to appreciate the need to have conversations about what is important to them at the end of life. As a result of this shift, death, dying and bereavement are becoming less taboo and more recognized as subjects to be discussed, explored and normalized within our society. Death will no longer be seen as a medical failure but rather as a normative life event.

Canadians are going to expect that their health-care providers be available to have discussions about advance care planning and will be able to support them as they navigate the decision-making required as we examine our options. But it won't just be up to our health-care system to support us. We are going to expect our families to be open to having discussions with us about our hopes, fears and needs at the end of life. We will also look to our education system to prepare not only our health-care providers but our children in order to increase our death literacy as a country.

Canadians will also have expectations that the organizations and corporations where we work will be places of compassion that make space for the acknowledgement of all the transitions associated with life and death. We will see our communities as playing an active role in caring for us and those we love as we transition from life to death. A compassionate community can empower the end-of-life experience for all Canadians.

As Canadians recognize that talking about death will not kill them, our relationship with death will change. We will begin to be able to develop an understanding of the dying process, our needs, our hopes and fears and create a more pervasive cultural support system that may ease the burden of dying on individuals. And just maybe we will begin to see that death isn't such a conversation-killer after all. Now go—get talking!

Resources

INTERNATIONAL

Aging with Dignity: Five Wishes: An American website to support advance care planning for older adults.

- https://www.agingwithdignity.org

Caring Bridge: An online platform that provides a simple health journaling tool that people who are ill can use to connect with their friends and families provide updates and receive support.

- https://www.caringbridge.org

The Conversation Project: Dedicated to helping people talk about their wishes for end-of-life care.

- http://theconversationproject.org

Dying Matters: A website bringing the conversation about death to the forefront.

- http://www.dyingmatters.org

eHospice: A globally run news and information resource committed to bringing you the latest news, commentary and analysis from the world of hospice, palliative and end-of-life care.

- http://www.ehospice.com

GeriPal: Focuses on palliative care for older individuals and the specific needs of geriatric patients and their providers.

- http://www.geripal.org

Get Palliative Care: An introduction to palliative care and the associated support services.

- https://getpalliativecare.org/blog/

PostHope: An online platform that allows people to create their own website to keep their family informed, and to receive donations and other offers of support and assistance throughout their illness.

- https://posthope.org/about

Prepare for Your Care: An American website developed by a geriatrician that helps you make informed decisions to get the care that is right for you.

- https://www.prepareforyourcare.org

CANADIAN

Best Endings: A website designed by patient advocate Kathy Kastner that curates material that makes end-of-life planning easier.

- https://www.bestendings.com/personal-decisions/

Canadian Hospice Palliative Care Association (CHPCA): Our national organization providing leadership and advocacy for quality hospice palliative care and increased awareness of end-of-life care issues.

- http://www.chpca.net

Canadian Virtual Hospice: Information and support on palliative and end-of-life care, loss and grief. A team of experts can answer your questions about life-threatening illness and loss.

- http://www.virtualhospice.ca

Family Caregiving for People at the End of Life: Website specifically organized to provide access to research, a range of relevant tools (including those developed through the research process), educational materials and networking opportunities for researchers, policymakers, decisionmakers, health-care professionals, related community organizations, individuals and families coping with caregiving issues.

- http://eolcaregiver.com

Living My Culture: Video series that shares the lived experience of 64 people from 11 cultures to help improve quality of life and care that is culturally safe and inclusive. Stories about traditions, rituals and spirituality, experiences of care, after death ceremonies and grief are shared in more than 600 video clips (available in 11 languages).

- http://livingmyculture.ca/culture/

MyGrief.ca: A free online resource to help people work through their grief from the comfort of their own home, at their own pace. It was developed by family members who have "been there" and grief experts to complement existing community resources and help address the lack of grief services in Canada. It is also an education tool for health-care providers.

- http://www.mygrief.ca

Quality End-of-Life Care Coalition of Canada: A group of over 36 national organizations concerned about quality end-of-life care for all Canadians.

- http://www.qelccc.ca

Speak Up: An awareness campaign offering information for individuals and their families, health-care professionals, community organizations, educators and researchers pertaining to advance care planning with information specific to each province and territory.

- http://www.advancecareplanning.ca

The Last Word: A blog and website that discusses how common major life events impact wills and estate law.

- https://thelastword.ca/blog/

The Way Forward: A website that outlines the path Hospice Palliative Care is taking to become fully integrated into communities and across all settings of care. Encourages Canadians to become involved in the process.

- http://hpcintegration.ca

GOVERNMENT OF CANADA

After a Death: Contains resources and information that can help you when someone dies. Links include first steps, obtaining a death certificate, what to cancel, possible benefits and managing finances.

- https://www.canada.ca/en/employment-social-development/services/benefits/family/death.html

Benefits for Parents of Critically Ill Children: Benefits paid to eligible parents who have to be away from work to provide care or support to their critically ill or injured child.

- https://www.canada.ca/en/services/benefits/ei/ei-critically-illchildren.html

Compassionate Care Benefits: An overview of the benefits available to eligible individuals requiring temporary leaves from work to provide care or support to a family member who is seriously or terminally ill or at end of life.

- https://www.canada.ca/en/employment-social-development/programs/ei/ei-list/reports/compassionate-care.html

End-of-Life Care: Information about end-of-life care, including palliative care and medical assistance in dying.

- https://www.canada.ca/en/health-canada/topics/end-life-care.html?_ga=1.267228878.1516425768.1426607858

Resource List: A list of palliative care links and publications covering various topics from caregiving and planning for end-of-life care to health research, policies, hospice palliative care directories, coalitions and education.

- https://www.canada.ca/en/health-canada/services/health-caresystem/palliative-end-life-care/resources.html

BRITISH COLUMBIA

Accessing End-of-life Care: Offers information about services that aim to preserve an individual's comfort, dignity and quality of life as their needs change, and to offer ongoing support for family and friends.

- http://www2.gov.bc.ca/gov/content/health/accessing-health-care/home-community-care/care-options-and-cost/end-of-life-care

B.C. Bereavement Helpline: A non-profit, free and confidential service that connects the public to grief support services within the province of B.C.

- 1-877-779-2223/1-604-738-9950

- http://www.bcbereavementhelpline.com

B.C. Centre for Palliative Care: An association of health-care experts providing leadership for best practice, research and education in palliative care, advance care planning and building compassionate communities.

- http://www.bc-cpc.ca/cpc/

B.C. Government Advance Care Planning: A website that helps to guide thinking about your beliefs, values and wishes regarding future health-care treatment.

- http://www2.gov.bc.ca/gov/content/family-social-supports/seniors/health-safety/advance-care-planning

B.C. Hospice Palliative Care Association: A not-for-profit membership organization committed to promoting and delivering hospice and palliative care to British Columbians.

- https://bchpca.org

Community Resources for Family Caregivers in B.C.: A list of references and information for caregivers and health professionals.

- https://www.doctorsofbc.ca/sites/default/files/resourcesforcaregivers-tearsheet.pdf

Expressing My Wishes for Future Health-Care Treatment Advance Care Planning Guide (PDF document): A guide and workbook to help people to complete an advance care plan that outlines wishes about healthcare decisions.

- http://www.health.gov.bc.ca/library/publications/year/2013/MyVoice-AdvanceCarePlanningGuide.pdf

Family Caregivers of B.C.: A registered non-profit dedicated to supporting family caregivers.

- http://www.familycaregiversbc.ca

ALBERTA

Advance Care Planning: A website that helps guide thinking about your beliefs, values and wishes regarding future health-care treatment.

- http://www.humanservices.alberta.ca/guardianship-trusteeship/personal-directives-how-it-works.html

Alberta Hospice Palliative Care Association: The provincial palliative care association for Alberta.

- http://www.ahpca.ca

Financial Support: Information provided by the Canadian Cancer Association that offers resources for benefits and financial support specific to Albertans.

- http://www.cancer.ca/en/support-and-services/support-services/financial-help-ab/?region=ab

Grief Support Program: Offers individual, family and group services.

- http://www.albertahealthservices.ca/info/facility.aspx?id=6&service=1026229

My Health Alberta: The Alberta Government and Alberta Health Services website with up-to-date information for Albertans about their health care.

- https://myhealth.alberta.ca/palliative-care

My Health Alberta Advance Care Planning: Advance Care planning information for Albertans.

- http://www.albertahealthservices.ca/info/page12585.aspx

Palliative Care: A website that offers links to palliative and end-of-life care resources.

- http://www.albertahealthservices.ca/info/Page14778.aspx

SASKATCHEWAN

Caring Hearts Camp: A weekend camp for children and teens who have recently experienced a loss due to the death of a family member or friend.

- http://www.rpci.org/caring-hearts-camp

My Voice—Advance Care Planning booklet (PDF): A workbook to provide you with the information you need to make informed choices about your future health care ahead of time.

- http://www.rqhealth.ca/rqhr-central-files/my-voice

Regina Palliative Care Inc.: Organization with a mandate to lead palliative and bereavement care for Saskatchewan through education, advocacy, counselling and support.

- http://www.rpci.org

Regina Qu'Appelle Health Region: Provides education on advance care planning in RQHR to both staff and the community.

- http://www.rqhealth.ca/department/advance-care-planning/advance-care-planning

Saskatchewan Government: Offers access to health-care directives and publications.

- http://www.publications.gov.sk.ca/details.cfm?p=77995

Saskatchewan Hospice Palliative Care Association: Advocates for hospice palliative care, including bereavement, through networking, education and research.

- http://www.saskpalliativecare.org

MANITOBA

Government of Manitoba: Palliative care and advance care planning information.

- https://www.gov.mb.ca/health/palliative_care.html

Health Care Directive: Advance care planning information for Manitobans.

- https://www.gov.mb.ca/health/livingwill.html

Palliative Manitoba: A registered charity that is focused on improving living until the end of life.

- http://palliativemanitoba.ca

Support for Grieving Children: Makes grief support services available to young people, helping them cope with grief that accompanies loss, and provides them with tools to deal with future emotions.

- http://palliativemanitoba.ca/programs-and-services/support-forgrieving-children/

YUKON AND NORTHWEST TERRITORIES

Home and Community Care: A service offering nursing care and support for personal care and daily living activities when people are no longer able to perform these activities on their own.

- http://www.hss.gov.nt.ca/en/services/continuing-care-services/ home-and-community-care

Hospice Yukon: Offers a range of bereavement and palliative support services with the vision of enhancing the quality of life for all people in the Yukon facing death and bereavement.

- http://www.hospiceyukon.net

Yukon Palliative Care Program: Provides clinical and psychosocial support to people in the Yukon living with a life-limiting illness and their families, with the goal of achieving the best possible quality of life until the end of life.

- http://www.hss.gov.yk.ca/palliativecare.php

ONTARIO

Bereaved Families of Ontario: Organization that dedicates its work to bereavement support through self-help and mutual aid. Programs are facilitated by trained volunteers who are themselves bereaved. Volunteer health professionals support our facilitators and advise programs.

- http://www.bereavedfamilies.net

CPR Decision Aids: Materials to help prepare individuals and their families for shared decision-making.

- http://speakupontario.ca/resource/cpr-decision-aids/

Hospice Palliative Care Ontario: A provincial association of hospices and palliative care providers, professionals and volunteers throughout Ontario. They envision a future where every person and family in the province of Ontario can quickly and easily access the finest standard of hospice palliative care when required.

- http://www.hpco.ca

Ontario Palliative Care Network: A partnership of community stakeholders, health service providers and health systems planners who are developing a coordinated and standardized approach for delivering hospice palliative care.

- http://www.ontariopalliativecarenetwork.ca/node/31841

Palliative Care Toolkit for Aboriginal Communities: Resource toolkit and reference material meant for First Nations, Métis and Inuit families and communities to help support individuals with cancer who have palliative care needs. These education materials can be used by anyone in the community.

- https://www.cancercareontario.ca/en/guidelines-advice/treatmentmodality/palliative-care/toolkit-aboriginal-communities

QUEBEC

Provincial Palliative Care Association: Offers a service to any person with a terminal illness who wants to spend their last days at home.

- http://www.societedesoinspalliatifs.com

NEW BRUNSWICK

Government Forms: Outlines advance care directives. It also includes legislation regarding advance care directives and a form to fill out.

- http://www2.gnb.ca/content/gnb/en/departments/health/patientinformation/content/advance_health_care_directives.html

Horizon Health Network: A healthcare services agency delivering palliative care services in English and French.

- http://en.horizonnb.ca/facilities-and-services/services/clinicalservices/palliative-care.aspx

Hospice Moncton: A registered charity promoting awareness and services to support those with life-limiting illnesses and their families.

- http://hospicemoncton.ca

New Brunswick Hospice Palliative Care Association: Provincial palliative care association.

- https://www.nbhpca-aspnb.ca

NOVA SCOTIA

Nova Scotia Palliative Care Association: A provincial body for hospice and palliative care in Nova Scotia.

- http://nshpca.ca

Personal Directives: Provides information for Nova Scotians regarding the Personal Directives Act.

- https://novascotia.ca/just/pda/

PRINCE EDWARD ISLAND

Advance Care Planning: Provincial advance care planning information.

- https://www.princeedwardisland.ca/en/information/health-pei/advance-care-planning

Health PEI: An overview of palliative care and how it can help an individual and their family. The website also provides contact information for further services and inquiries.

- https://www.princeedwardisland.ca/en/information/health-pei/palliative-care-program?utm_source=redirect&utm_medium=url&utm_campaign=palliative-care

Hospice PEI: A volunteer-driven organization assisting people in PEI by preparing, supporting and caring for those affected by a life-limiting illness before and after death.

- https://www.hospicepei.com

NEWFOUNDLAND

Newfoundland Palliative Care Association: Strives to provide leadership in palliative care in Newfoundland

and Labrador advocating for holistic palliative care to enhance the quality of life.

- https://www.nlpalliativecareassociation.net

Examples of Compassionate Community Initiatives

CANADA

B.C. Centre for Palliative Care: Outlines the efforts the centre is making to promote compassionate community initiatives throughout the province of British Columbia.

- http://www.bc-cpc.ca/cpc/compassionate-communities/

Carpenter Hospice: Tools this community group is using to develop their compassionate communities initiatives.

- https://www.thecarpenterhospice.com/resources/compassionatecity-charter/compassionate-city-charter-3c-tools/

Hospice Northwest: Die-alogues: A community-driven initiative providing opportunities for people to join together and learn about and discuss dying, death, loss and bereavement.

- https://www.hospicenorthwest.ca/how-we-can-help/die-alogues/

Windsor-Essex Compassion Care Community: How the community of Windsor-Essex is working together to improve quality of living and care for their citizens.

- http://compassionatecarecommunity.com

INTERNATIONAL

The GroundSwell Project (Australia): Organization working to normalize and socialize dying, death, loss and bereavement.

- http://www.thegroundswellproject.com

England: An overview of some initiatives in the U.K. (PDF document).

- http://www.compassionatecommunities.org.uk/files/PDF/CC_Report_Final_July_2013-2.pdf

New Health Foundation (Spain): A self-described social awareness program leading compassionate community initiatives in Spain.

- http://www.newhealthfoundation.org/en/community/

Public Health Palliative Care International: An international association leading the compassionate communities movement.

- http://www.phpci.info

Acknowledgements

Writing this book did not kill me! I am very thankful to all those who ensured that I survived relatively unscathed.

To the dynamic team at ECW Press: Susan Renouf, my patient and wise editor, Rachel Ironstone, Jessica Albert, Jen Knoch and Crissy Calhoun—thank you for believing that these are indeed essential conversations. Much gratitude is owed my savvy and lovely agent at Transatlantic, Jesse Finkelstein, for truly understanding that how we die matters and for taking a chance on me. Thank you to Alexia Vernon for helping me to develop the original book proposal and always encouraging me with moxie. My birthday twin Susan Goldberg graciously provided invaluable edits early on in the writing process that allowed me to focus my ideas. Thank you for letting me lean on you.

I am incredibly grateful to be a part of the dynamic hospice palliative care community that continues to grow and improve how Canadians live until they die. It is the leadership of groups like the Canadian Hospice Palliative Care Association and Hospice Palliative Care Ontario that moves this work forward and helps us all to normalize and socialize dying, death, loss and bereavement. Thank you to all my palliative care mentors, friends and colleagues who have supported my work and made me feel like I have something to contribute.

Thank you to my family and friends who have supported me along the way. I'm incredibly blessed to be so well loved and encouraged. Much love to my husband, Kevin, who put up with me being extra distracted and was always there with loving reassurance and a willingness to read a section. And of course our children, Allegra and Dawson, who probably think they are growing up in a home where we *only* talk about dying and death and yet somehow we manage to be really enjoying life, too.

Selected Bibliography

Abel, J., Bowra, J., Walter, T., & Howarth, G. (2011). Compassionate community networks: supporting home dying. *BMJ Supportive & Palliative Care,* 1(2), 129–33.

Ariès, P. (1982). *The hour of our death.* Vintage.

Attig, T. (2010). *How we grieve: Relearning the world.* Oxford University Press.

Back, A.L., Arnold, R.M., & Quill, T.E. (2003). Hope for the best, and prepare for the worst. *Annals of Internal Medicine, 138* (5), 439–43.

Beahm, G. (Ed.). (2011). *I, Steve: Steve Jobs in his own words.* Agate Publishing.

Brubaker, J.R., Hayes, G.R., & Dourish, P. (2013). Beyond the grave: Facebook as a site for the expansion of death and mourning. *The Information Society, 29* (3), 152–63.

Byock, I., & Byock, A. (1997). *Dying well: The prospect for growth at the end of life.* New York: Riverhead Books.

Byock, I. (1998). *Dying well.* Penguin.

Byock, I. (2012). *The best care possible.* New York: Avery.

Callahan, D. (2000). *The troubled dream of life: In search of a peaceful death.* Georgetown University Press.

Canadian Hospice Palliative Care Association: http://www.chpca.net.

Chochinov, H.M. (2007). Dignity and the essence of medicine: The A, B, C, and D of dignity conserving care. *BMJ: British Medical Journal 335* (7612), 184.

Chochinov, H.M. (2012). *Dignity therapy: Final words for final days.* OUP USA.

CHPCA Compassionate Companies: http://www.chpca.net/news-andevents/backgrounder-canadian-compassionate-companies.aspx, http://www.chpca.net/media/351526/Compassionate_Companies_Research_Update.pdf.

College of Physicians and Surgeons of Ontario FAQ on MAID: http://www.cpso.on.ca/CPSO/media/documents/Policies/Policy-Items/medical-assistance-in-dying-FAQ.pdf?ext=.pdf.

DeSpelder, L.A., & Strickland, A.L. (1996). *The last dance: Encountering death and dying.* Houston: Mayfield Publishing Co.

Gawande, A. (2014). *Being mortal: Medicine and what matters in the end.* Metropolitan Books.

Getty, E., Cobb, J., Gabeler, M., Nelson, C., Weng, E., & Hancock, J. (2011). I said your name in an empty room: Grieving and continuing bonds on Facebook. In *Proceedings of the SIGCHI Conference on human factors in computing systems* (997–1000). ACM.

Gibbs, M., Meese, J., Arnold, M., Nansen, B., & Carter, M. (2015). #Funeral and Instagram: Death, social media, and platform vernacular. *Information, Communication & Society, 18* (3), 255–68.

Gordon, A.K., & Klass, D. (1979). *They need to know: How to teach children about death.* New Jersey: Prentice Hall.

Granger, K. (2013). Healthcare staff must properly introduce themselves to patients. *BMJ: British Medical Journal (Online),* 347.

Granger, K. (2014). Death by social networking: The rising prominence of social media in the palliative care setting. *BMJ Supportive & Palliative Care 4* (1), 2–3.

Grollman., E.A. (1991). *Talking about death: A dialogue between parent and child.* Beacon Press.

Harpham, W.S. (2011). *When a parent has cancer: A guide to caring for your children.* Harper Collins.

Hello My Name Is: https://hellomynameis.org.uk.

Kalish, R.A. (1985). The social context of death and dying. *Handbook of aging and the social sciences, 2,* 149–70.

Kellehear, A. (2005). *Compassionate cities: Public health and end-of-life care.* London: Routledge.

Kellehear, A. (2013). Compassionate communities: End-of-life care as everyone's responsibility. *QJM: An International Journal of Medicine, 106* (12), 1071–5.

Key facts about carers. (2013). Carers Trust: www.carers.org/key-factsabout-carers.

Kübler-Ross, E. (2009). *On death and dying: What the dying have to teach doctors, nurses, clergy and their own families.* Taylor & Francis.

Kylmä, J., Duggleby, W., Cooper, D., & Molander, G. (2009). Hope in palliative care: An integrative review. *Palliative & Supportive Care, 7* (3), 365–77.

Larkin, P.J. (2016). Can compassion transform our dying? A reading of compassion for palliative and end-of-life care. *Journal for the Study of Spirituality, 6* (2), 168–79.

Maciel, C., & Pereira, V.C. (Eds.). (2013). *Digital legacy and interaction: Post-mortem issues.* Springer Science & Business Media.

Martin, S. (2016). *A good death.* Toronto: Harper Collins

Medical Assistance in Dying: https://www.canada.ca/en/health-canada/services/medical-assistance-dying.html.

National Council for Palliative Care. (2013). *Who cares? Support for carers of people approaching the end of life.* http://www.ncpc.org.uk/sites/default/files/Who_Cares_Conference_Report.pdf.

Noonan, K., Horsfall, D., Leonard, R., & Rosenberg, J. (2016). Developing death literacy. *Progress in Palliative Care, 24* (1), 31–5.

Northcott, H.C., & Wilson, D.M. (2016). *Dying and death in Canada.* University of Toronto Press.

Nuland, S.B. (1994). *How we die: Reflections on life's final chapter.* Vintage.

Papadatou, D., & Papadatos, C.J. (Eds.). (1991). *Children and death.* Taylor & Francis.

Paul-Choudhury, S. (2011). Digital legacy: The fate of your online soul. *New Scientist, 210* (2809), 41–3.

Plett, Heather: http://heatherplett.com/2015/03/hold-space/.

Public Health Palliative Care International: http://www.phpci.info.

Ratner, E.R., & Song, J.Y. (2002). Education for the end of life. *Chronicle of Higher Education, 48* (39), B12.

Sacks, O. (2015). *Gratitude.* Knopf Canada.

Saul, P. (2015) TEDx talk: Let's talk about dying (video file): https://www.youtube.com/watch?v=bJ7rCIq9Lc0.

Saunders, D.C.M. (2006). *Cicely Saunders: Selected writings 1958–2004.* Oxford University Press.

Steinhauser, K.E., Christakis, N.A., Clipp, E.C., McNeilly, M., McIntyre, L., & Tulsky, J.A. (2000). Factors considered important at the end of life by patients, family, physicians, and other care providers. *Jama, 284* (19), 2476–82.

Steinhauser, K.E., Clipp, E.C., McNeilly, M., Christakis, N.A., McIntyre, L.M., & Tulsky, J.A. (2000). In search of a good death: Observations of patients, families, and providers. *Annals of Internal Medicine, 132* (10), 825–32.

Stowe, H.B. (1888). *Little Foxes.* Houghton, Mifflin.

Taylor, C. (2017). *Dying: A memoir.* Tin House Books.

Taubert, M., Watts, G., Boland, J., & Radbruch, L. (2014). Palliative social media. *BMJ Supportive & Palliative Care, 4* (1), 13–18.

Thompson, N., & Lund, D.A. (2017). *Loss, grief, and trauma in the workplace.* Routledge.

Wee, B. (2016). Ambitions for palliative and end-of-life care. *Clinical Medicine, 16* (3), 213–4.

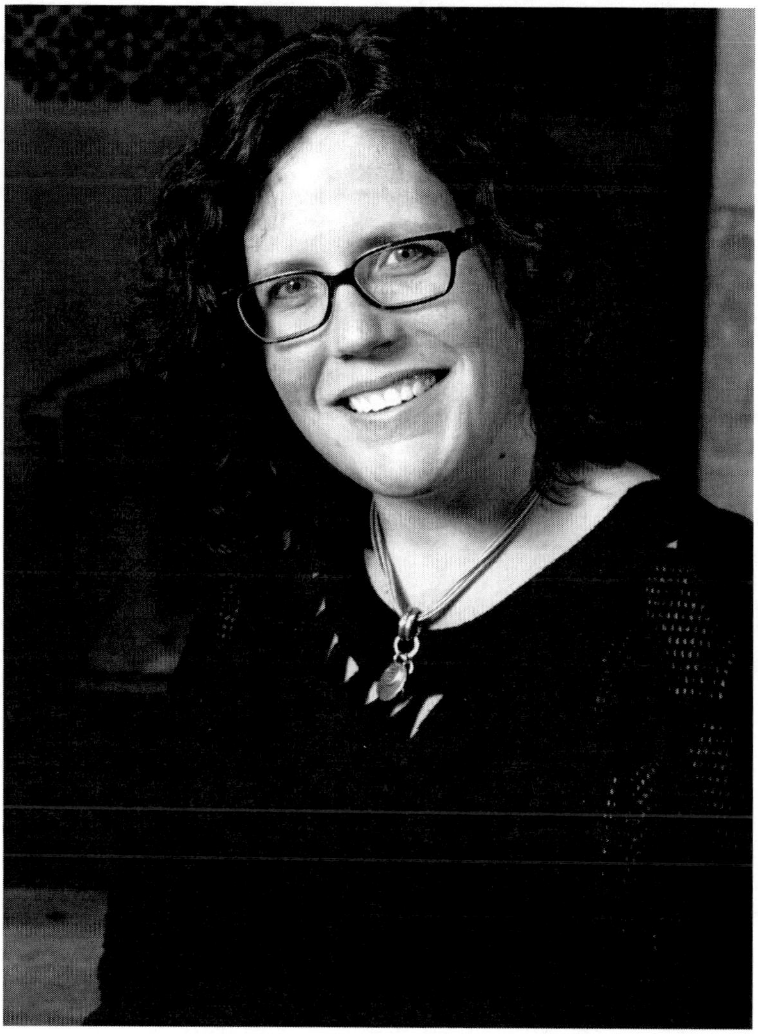

Dr. Kathy Kortes-Miller is an assistant professor at the School of Social Work and the Palliative Care Division Lead at the Centre for Education and Research on Aging and Health (CERAH) at Lakehead University. She is an unconventional death educator with a passion for palliative care and improving end-of-life care for all.

Back Cover Material

"Practical, compassionate, wise ... Kortes-Miller's examples illuminate her most telling points, and their authenticity is palpable, as they are drawn from her own experiences."

Phil Dwyer, author of *Conversations on Dying*

"It's hard to imagine a better guide to end-of-life conversations ... I especially welcomed her consideration of the role played by social media in death and mourning."

Katherine Ashenburg, author of *The Mourner's Dance*

"From conversation starters to suggestions on what questions to ask, this book will help people and families navigate toward a good death and, ultimately, a good life."

Ian Bos, activist and cross-Canada walker for Hospice Palliative Care

"With insights born of her commitment to her profession, Kathy Kortes-Miller gives readers concrete strategies when facing life's end. Rather than preaching, she empowers both patients and caregivers with questions that help focus on strengths."

Kathy Kastner, blogger at BestEndings.com and author of *Death Kills ... and other things I've learned on the internet*

Noted palliative–care educator and researcher Dr. Kathy Kortes-Miller shows how to identify and reframe limiting beliefs about dying. With humour and compassion, she addresses topics such as

- advance care plans
- how to have conversations about end-of-life wishes
- how to manage challenging family dynamics
- how to talk to children about death
- how to build a compassionate workplace
- practical strategies to supporting our colleagues
- how to talk to health-care practitioners
- medical assistance in dying (MAID)

Far from morbid, these conversations are full of meaning and life – and the relief that comes from knowing what your loved ones want, and what you want for yourself. *Talking About Death Won't Kill You* is the essential handbook to help individuals navigate personal and medical decisions for the best quality of-life for the end of our lives.

G

H

K

L

M

T

U

V

W

Made in United States
North Haven, CT
05 November 2026

21768318R10143